Spiritual Medicine

A Trilogy
of
Thinking, Feeling and Willing

Third edition 2020

*Understood through
Anthroposophy, Demonology and Christology.*

By

Are Simeon Thoresen DVM
Margaret Mary Fleming DVM, AP

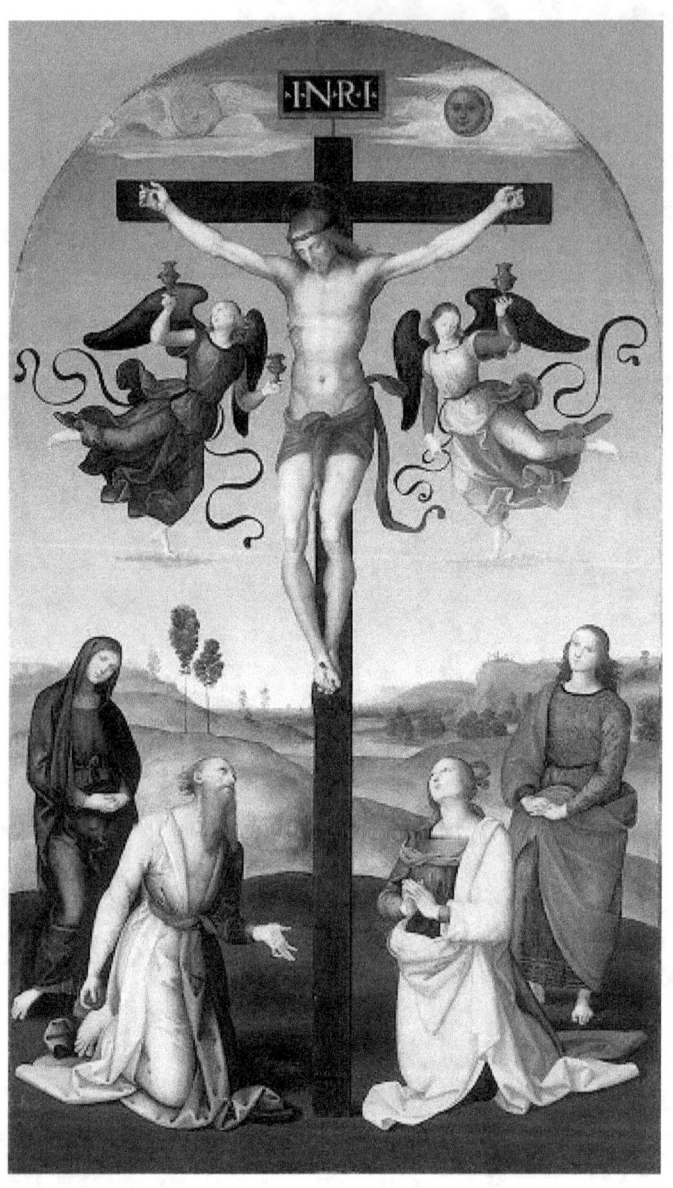

© 2018 Are Simeon Thoresen, DVM

For questions on the rights of this book please contact:

Are Thoresen
Leikvollgata 31
N-3213 Sandefjord
Email: arethore@online.no

All rights reserved. The contents of this book, both photographic and textual, may not be reproduced in any form; by print, photo print, photo transparency, microfilm, microfiche, slide or any other means, nor may it be included in any computer retrieval system without written permission from the publisher.

Remark: The author takes no responsibility for the practical use of the methods described in this book.

This book aims to give readers, professional and lay, an understanding of the *spiritual* foundations of alternative medicine, philosophy, principles and practice.

Printed version;   **ISBN 9781986236973**

Published by Are Thoresen

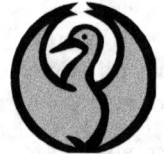

*Dedicated to All
Who Seek to Heal and Understand*

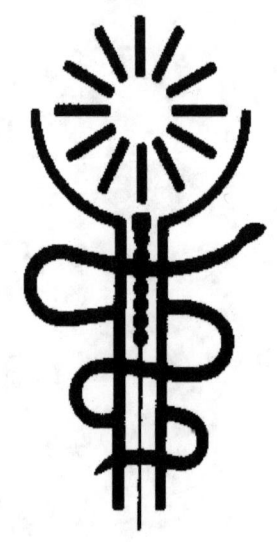

Important foreword
***

Dear reader.

This book is the black/white edition of „Spiritual Healing", written in cooperation by me, Are Thoresen, and my colleague Margareth Fleming.

As with all conscious and old souls, we soon disagreed on several things, among other such a simple thing whether to print the book in black/white or colors, the last option causing the book to be considerably more expensive.

We decided then to publish two versions of the book, one in black/white, sort of a „my" version, and one in color, sort of „her" version.

During the time that has passed since the time of publishing, I have passed through a deep and radical development within medicine and healing, so deep and radical that the book needs an update.

The development concerns mainly the phenomenon of translocation of diseases, as described and discussed in the four books I have published since „Spiritual Medicine" emerged.

These four books are:
- „Translocation" (autumn 2019)
- „Acupuncture and Translocation" (autumn 2019)
- „Spirituality and Translocation" (spring 2020)
- „5000 years of Deceit, the Yellow Emperor Unveiled" (autumn 2020)

As this development and change just relate to my (Ares) insights, and not to Margareths, I chose to update only the black/white version, and leave the color version intact, as it has been.

The color version will as such be even more Margareths, and the black/white version will be even more mine.

I hope the readers can live with this split.

I thus welcome the readers to a new and deeper experience of the black/white version of „Spiritual Medicine".

Sandefjord, 11th of February 2020

Yours sincerely

Are Thoresen

Contents

Part One of the Trilogy: *Anthroposophy.*
The 7- and 19 parts Way to Therapy.
The Faculty of Thinking.

Part Two of the Trilogy: *Demonology.*
Demons.
Translocation of diseases, transformation.
The Faculty of Feeling.

Part Three of the Trilogy: *Christology.*
The Middle Point and the Group.
The Christ-force.
The transformation of the 5-elements to 12-elements.
The correction of the pulse-positions
The Faculty of Willing.

Prologue

Phil Rogers D.V.M.

Many people will be upset greatly by three words - Demons, Spiritual and Christology - in the title of this book. These words will cause many others to question the sanity of the author, Are Simeon Thoresen.

Psychic ability – the Sixth Sense – is a primitive sense inherent in all living things. Its basic purpose in animals and people is to aid survival, viz to sense danger, find water, food, shelter, missing young etc. Because urbanized people have lost touch with nature to a great extent, their physic sense has atrophied through lack of use. But it is still there and can be cultivated / rekindled by proper training.

Genius is a rare commodity that few of us attain. I see the color-magic painted by Van Gogh, hear the music-magic of Beethoven, imagine touching the exquisite bronze of Rodin's Thinker. I revere their work but know that I can never create such beauty. As it is with Are's psychic skills.

Are has been a friend for more than 20 years. My initial impressions were that he was either a con-man, or mentally deluded, living in a world of make-believe. However, having spent time with him, seeing him work, talking to some of his human patients and animal owners and reading his papers and books on healing, I now see him as a man of many talents, a veterinary colleague, acupuncturist, homeopath, naturopath, psychic, Seer, gifted healer and seeker-of-truth.

Stress is at record levels today. Rates of marriage breakup, antisocial behavior, mental disorders, psychoactive medication, drug addiction, alcoholism, criminality, self-harm and suicide are very high. Could this be because many people do not believe in a Supreme God, the Great Healer and Creator of all that exists?

Could this be because they deny the possibility of evil discarnate Spirits invading their body-mind-Spirit?

Non-believers deny the reality of an afterlife, viz that the human soul/Spirit are immortal. They may accept that Jesus Christ was a great teacher but deny that he was the God-Essence in human form. They do not believe in Angels or Demons. Such people are unlikely to read this book. That will be their loss, for there is much to learn about themselves and their physical, mental and Spiritual health within these pages.

We all have our individual strengths and weaknesses.

We all harbor Dark Passengers to some extent. Few will master Are's ability to See / sense the Spirit World as he does. But if you are a thinker and seeker-of-truth, I urge you to read this book and to try his methods. Some of them may work for you. If you have serious health issues, especially mental / Spiritual issues, put your trust in the infinite love of the Creator / Great Healer / Christ-Essence. Believe that those Almighty Powers can release your Demons.

So be it!

Phil Rogers, Dublin, Ireland
August 22
2016

The Journey

"With This book, I will take you on a journey......

A journey from medical school through acupuncture, homeopathy, and Anthroposophic medicine to Christianity.

A journey from symptomatic treatment to healing through grace and communion.

A journey from treating the material symptom, the energetic symptom and the etheric deficiency to evoking the free etheric energy of the middle, through the Christ point.

A journey to use the group to heal and transform the pathological demonic structures from disease to health.

A journey from causing the pathological entities to translocate to causing them to transform.

A journey from the head, where the energy for pulse findings first originated for me, and after 30 years of practice and meditation to the heart.

A journey from calculating after the 5 elements to calculate from the 12 etheric streams of the zodiac, the 12-element thinking.

In doing this, the ability to diagnose with the pulse is transformed to an ability to diagnose with the heart. As a result of this evolution, the effect of treatment is moved from the meridian system, which lies between the physical and etheric body, to the etheric body itself. As the etheric energy belongs wholly to the etheric body, there is a quantum leap in the development of the practitioner. That is why the effect and abilities of the physician may suddenly and fundamentally change.

This happened to my cancer treatment in 2014. Now to….

A journey from the restricted energy of the single individual, to the vast and unending energy of the group, of humanity.

A journey from the individual microcosm to the macrocosm of the group, and as such, the entire universe.

A journey from a binary system to that of a trinity.

A journey from Lucifer and Ahriman to Christ.

A journey in unveiling the teachings of the yellow emperor as a disguised teaching of Lucifer himself.

To be blessed by experiencing such a transition and journey is rare.

Those unprepared individuals who are dragged into such transformations are often left highly frustrated to the point of insanity, to the edge of suicide.

This is my journey….."

Of utmost importance

Today the knowledge and insight of the Spiritual World is vanishing rapidly as materialism takes its hold. Fewer and fewer people believe in God. Respect for other life forms, trees and animals as well as for non-material Beings has lessened, and egoistic materialism is progressing.

The culture is trembling under the weight of ignorance, and from where I stand I cannot see any rescue or salvation.

Our culture will vanish as all other cultures have vanished, and the cause of our destruction will be the ever-progressing materialism and egoism, that will eventually culminate in a "war of all against all".

The knowledge presented in this book along with all other similar knowledge will be carried over to the next culture by a small number of people who have grasped the need for Spirituality, and together they will create a new culture of Spiritual and Brotherly love.

Introduction

For the past twenty years I was haunted by my inability to truly obtain a sustainable cure in my patients. I observed that symptoms, rather than being annihilated, where being transferred. I named this phenomena "Translocation". Furthermore, I came to realize, as a result of my spiritual development, the reason for this translocation was the result of the free will of entities that actually reflect the symptomatology of the disease.

When I wrote the book "Demons, Spiritual Medicine"[1] in 2016-2018, I became increasingly aware of the importance of three major factors for transforming these entities and thus curing chronic disease and avoid translocation within the body or to other humans or animals. As was eluded to in the preface, I concluded that:

- first, one must treat a specific point on the patient's midsection dubbed "the Middle". This creates both a medical and a spiritual effect.
- Secondly one must treat the transforming forces of the pathological forces, and these transforming forces are to be found according the etheric streams of the zodiac, called the 12-elements, in a 90^0 angle (explained in detail later). This creates a medical effect.
- Thirdly, to also induce a more spiritual change in the patient, the middle-treatment should be performed in a group of people. Such a treatment creates a much deeper spiritual effect, although not necessarily a medical effect and change.

---

[1]Demons, Spiritual Medicine", Temple Lodge 2018

I also concluded that most forms of medicine, both conventional and alternative, are also dealing with the translocation process. Most therapists have no knowledge of the presence of these dynamic entities and would not recognize this obstacle to a true cure. As with my own experiences, I believe that these practitioners are also mostly transferring these pathological entities to other areas of the body and even other patients, both man and animals.

If one reviews the literature of various alternative medical systems, there are revelations that show that this translocation phenomena was already being observed, especially by some of the great physicians of homeopathy, such as Dr. Constantine Hering[2], the author of Hering's Laws of Cure.[3] The gold standard of the evidence of a cure was eloquently categorized by this physician as a centrifugal exteriorization of the symptoms from serious spiritual and organic disease to superficial areas such as the skin. The eventual positive outcome being a person with total

---

[2] Dr. Constantine Hering M.D. (1800 1880). Dr. Hering is aptly called the 'Father of Homoeopathy' in America. Originally a skeptic of homeopathy, he was convinced of its efficacy after an objective study of its principles. He went on to expound upon the Laws of cure.

[3] Herings Law of Cure. This law states that cure occurs from; a). From above and downwards. b). From within outwards. c). Appearance of symptoms in reverse chronological order. This means: a); "From above downwards." Cure progresses from the head towards the lower trunk, that is to say the head symptoms clear first. With regard to the extremities, cure spreads from shoulder to fingers, or hip to toes. b); Cure starts from within outwards. Cure progresses from more important organs (e.g. liver, endocrine) to less important organs (e.g. joints). That is to say, the function of vital organs are restored before those less important to life. The end result of this externalization of disease is often the production of "treatment cutaneous rash". c); "Appearance of symptoms in reverse chronological order". More recent symptoms and pathology will clear before old, the disease "back tracks" so to speak.

freedom of body, mind, and spirit in order to enlist his higher calling. What was not overtly addressed in this law was the transmission of such demons to other beings on the planet. Therefore, in a global perspective, this does not represent a cure.

The Acupuncture Method to Avoid Translocation

The only two methods I have found to avoid translocation and induce a true transformation came from the advice of Judith von Halle[4]. She told me that I must treat the patient using "Christ-Consciousness". Two methods can lead from such a consciousness to a therapeutic point, and that is:

- "the Middle point",
- "the 90^0-point".

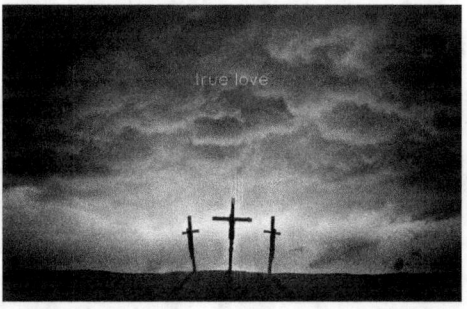

---

[4] Judith von Halle was born 1972 in Berlin. She is an architect by profession and has worked as such. She has felt herself to be especially bound to Christ since childhood. She encountered anthroposophy in 1997 and worked part time for the German Anthroposophical Society until 2005. From 2001 till 2003 she gave lectures in the Rudolf Steiner House about esoteric Judaism and the Apocalypse of St. John. During Easter 2004 the stigmata of Christ appeared on her. Since that happened she has only been able to consume water and abstained from solid nourishment.

The middle point as related to the anatomical middle

The spiritual depiction of the middle point as Christ is depicted in the above painting. Jesus Christ is positioned in the middle of two other robbers being similarly punished for their crimes.

The criminal to the right of Christ (representing Ahriman) mocked him and, as a result, was sentenced to eternal damnation, while the other criminal (representing Lucifer) begged to be saved and to enter the kingdom of heaven. Jesus told him that one day his wish would be granted.

The 90^0-point as related to the zodiac

This method is derived from the teachings of Rudolf Steiner about the effect of the morning-evening forces as opposed to the midday-midnight-forces[5].

> *From the East an endeavor will be made to strengthen what I have already explained: to place in the service of the earth the beings which work in from the opposite side of the cosmos. In the future there will be a great battle. Human science will stretch out to the cosmic, but will try to get there by different paths. It will be the task of good, healing science to find certain cosmic forces which can reach the earth through the co-operation of two cosmic streams, those of Pisces and Virgo. The great secret to be discovered will be how the influence which works from the direction of Pisces as a power of the sun unites itself with the influence working from the direction of Virgo. It will make for good when it is learnt how the morning and*

---

[5] «Reappearance of Christ in the Etheric", lecture 12, held on the 25th of November 1917, by Rudolf Steiner, GA 178.

evening forces from the two sides of the cosmos can be brought into the service of humanity.

These forces, however, will be left aside by those who try to achieve their whole purpose through the polaric duality of positive and negative forces. The forces which enable the spiritual to stream down to earth with the aid of positive and negative magnetism come from Gemini; they are the midday forces. In ancient times it was known that cosmic influences were involved in this, and to-day even exoteric scientists are aware that in some or other way positive and negative magnetism lie behind Gemini in the Zodiac. The aim will be to paralyze all that could be gained through a revelation of the true duality in the cosmos — to paralyze it in a materialistic, egotistic way by means of the forces which stream in particularly from Gemini and can be placed entirely at the service of the human "Double."

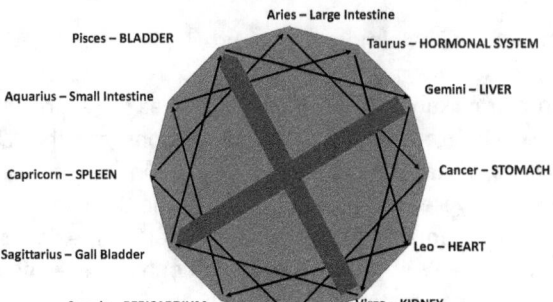

The 12 organs related to morning-evening forces

Aries – Large Intestine
Pisces – BLADDER
Taurus – HORMONAL SYSTEM
Aquarius – Small Intestine
Gemini – LIVER
Capricorn – SPLEEN
Cancer – STOMACH
Sagittarius – Gall Bladder
Leo – HEART
Scorpio – PERICARDIUM
Virgo – KIDNEY
Libra – LUNG

The first time I attempted to treat the middle point was on a horse during a veterinary course in Germany. I clearly saw, with my spiritual eyes, an ahrimanic pathological structure in the region of the abdomen, and a luciferic pathological structure in the region of the chest[6] Using my spiritual vision, I could also locate the middle point. My first attempt to treat this point was using an air gun called a dermojet to inject a small amount of B_{12} into the point. Quite to my surprise, instead of transforming and releasing them, these demons appeared to pull back. A participant in the course claimed that he saw them retract to the lower limbs.

From this observation, I realized that the middle point has a kind of "life force" of its own and, as such, requires the gentler treatment of an acupuncture needle or even one's fingers. In contrast, a dermojet forces fluid into the point by a forceful thrust of pressurized air. Electrical stimulators, magnetic wave generators and even cold lasers, are also ineffective and even deleterious in treating the Christ point. This is due to the fact that luciferic and ahrimanic elemental entities thrive off of these types of devices. I also learned that the transformational process is more complex than I realized. Despite the transformational process from virulent to benign, the latter structures remained. I came to

---

[6]The luciferic structures are almost always proximal or cranial. The ahrimanic structures are almost always distal or caudal. There is also another group of pathological structures, known in ancient tradition as the azuric demons. They are said to be a special group of the ahrimanic demons, and they attack the "I" itself of human beings. They are the most dangerous in the future in contrast to luciferic demons who were the most notorious of the three in former times. In our present time, the ahrimanic are the most malevolent. I seldom see the later, so there is not much I can say about them. Traditionally, the luciferic structure, relate to the feelings, or astral forces of the body, while the ahrimanic structure, relates to the growth or etheric forces. Traditionally the azuric structures or demons relate to the Spirit, the consciousness, the "I" organization of the body.

understand that, in actuality, man needs these entities in order to function in the material world. However, it is equally important that they remain a certain distance from each other while inhabiting the human form. If they get close enough to join forces, serious pathology can ensue. This will be discussed in detail in the second part of the trilogy entitled Demons.

Since 2014, I have treated many human and veterinary patients with the middle point, that is as single patients and not in a group, using one needle carefully placed in the middle, or with my fingers held in a gesture as shown in the picture below. Most patients seem to be satisfied with the effect of this treatment. Some patients actually describe an intense feeling of healing energy radiating throughout their bodies. I can see these patterns stream in the shape of a figure eight. Furthermore, my spiritual eye has observed that this healing energy will gravitate to the area of the body containing the demonic structure.

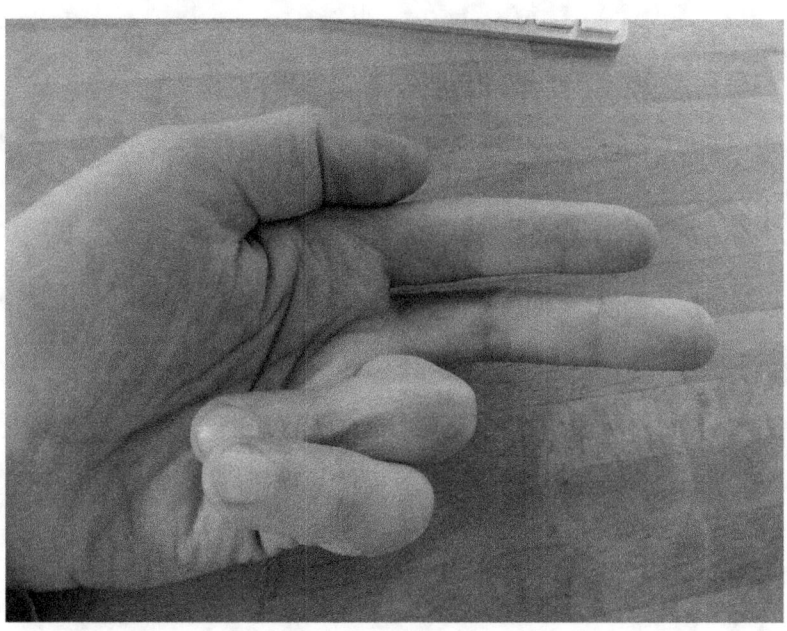

Unfortunately, I also started to discover that the positive effect I was seeing in so many patients was not happening in the very important disease of cancer.

In 2019 I added the method of the 90^0-system, and have since then treated every patient with both the anatomical middle and with the points revealed through the 90^0-force zodiacal method.

This combination has given the best results, also relating to the curing effect in cancer.

Spiritual Medicine

Part One

Three-fold way to

Therapy

The Faculty of Thinking

Anthroposophy.

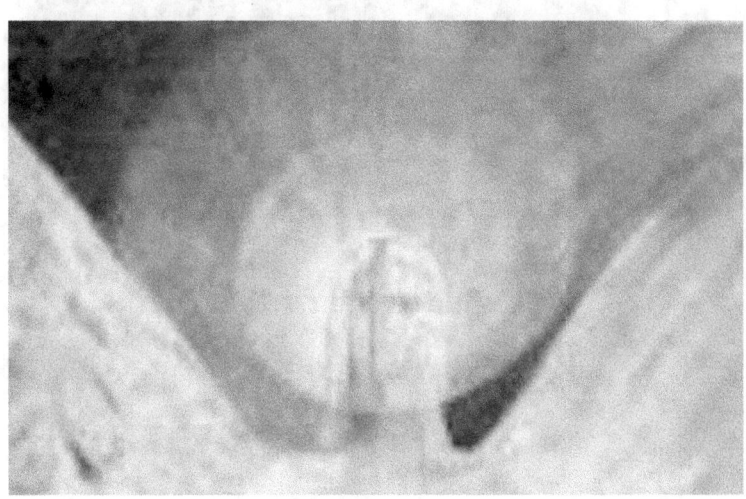

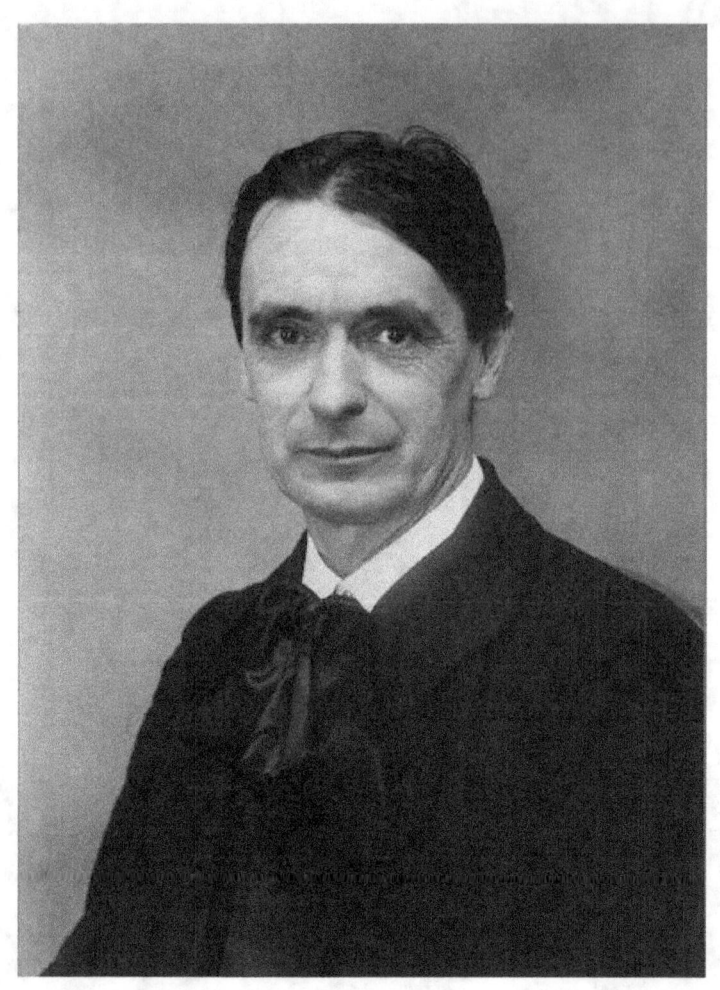

Rudolf Steiner

(Father of Anthroposophy)

Chapter 1

My first book, "Holistic Veterinary Medicine", was written in 1986. During the years from 1986, until now, I have gone through a deep development with many realizations, spiritually, energetically, religiously and professionally.

I have come to the insight that all disease is caused by the presence of spiritual pathological structures that are either of a Luciferic or Ahrimanic nature. They can develop from or come from:

- the already excising human Luciferic part, which is a part of our substantiality
- the already excising human Ahrimanic part, which is a part of our substantiality
- Or they can come from other human beings as "free" demonic forces, and may be called "demons"

These structures may have an etheric structure (body), an astral structure (body) or even an "I"-like structure (body), but no 'I' as such (implying an absence of moral code)[7]. These structures cause

---

[7] Steiner believed that the human body is made up of 4 sheaths. The first is the physical body of substances gathered from (and that return to) the inorganic world. The second layer is the life force also called the etheric body, in common with all living creatures, including plants. It provides the living formative forces that sculpt the individual physical body. This etheric body is closely connected to its physical counterpart and stays with it during sleep and death. The third layer is termed the astral body and relates to consciousness, in common with all animals. It consists of soul forces which are living forces that fine tune the physical. The astral body contains the senses and is the instrument of emotions and feelings. Finally, the fourth layer called the "I" is the ego which anchors the faculty of self-awareness and free will unique to human beings. It is associated with the spirit, a substrate that is higher than the soul. The "I" conveys divine

disease, and through both alternative and traditional treatment, they can easily be transferred to other parts of the body or to other living creatures, especially animals. The transformation of these entities can, to my knowledge and experience, be done only through the power and consciousness of Christ.

There are 3 types of demons.

In the spiritual world on the other side of the threshold, there are many kinds of entities, just as in the physical world. Here in the physical world, we may meet innumerable types of beings, some are beneficial to us, some are indifferent and some are dangerous. In the spiritual world it is just as in the physical world, and those beings or entities that are dangerous to us we call "adversaries".

There are many different types of these adversaries, but to make it easier to define them we may divide them into three groups:

- the ahrimanic beings, "demons or ahrimanic demons", which are ahrimanic adversarial entities in the etheric realm, which want us to be more materialistic and deny the spiritual world.
- the luciferic beings, "specters or luciferic demons", which are luciferic adversarial entities in the astral realm, which want us to lose ourselves in our own subjective experiences of the spiritual world.
- the azuric beings, "phantoms or azuric demons", which are azuric adversarial entities in both the physical and spiritual realms, attacking the physical body as well as the "I" or "I

---

human selfhood that gives us the capacity for transformation. Both the astral and I body can separate from the physical and etheric during sleep and after death. The 'I' is immortal and reincarnates.

organization", who want us to lose our "I", or make the "I" egoistic and unsuitable for the spiritual world.

I mentioned earlier that if we are not conscious inside our separated soul parts with our awakened "I", then alien and malignant forces have the possibility of entering our being. A meeting with these powers, internal or external, seems to be inevitable when working with crossing the threshold and passing into the spiritual world.

The hands as spiritual sensory organs.

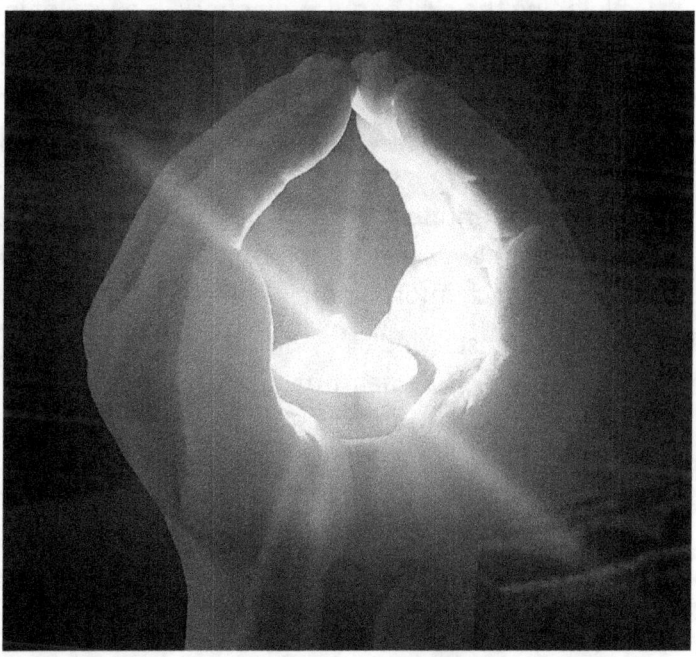

The hands are highly spiritual organs. They can, when the fingertips meet the blood, as in acupuncture pulse diagnosis[8], be transformed to highways into the spiritual world. They serve as organs of initiation (an anthroposophic term describing the process of being initiated into the spirit world, discussed later in this chapter). The pulse-diagnosis that I use to diagnose my acupuncture patients is not a technique; it is a state of consciousness. The changes in the pulse are not happening physically, but spiritually. To be able to detect pulse changes, we must be in that spiritual world. To enter it, we have to separate our thinking, feeling, and willing (This important spiritual trinity will be explained in more detail throughout this book), or as described as the "Northern way", the etheric body from the astral body. Developing the skill of pulse-diagnosis is a way of initiation into that consciousness.

I have also discovered that most diseases (>90%) in children and animals are projections (translocations) from adults, especially the parents and/or owners. Furthermore, these projections are living pathological entities, or, In other words, "demons". All symptoms are simply an expression of disease as "pathological" information, and such information is not lost.

In Traditional Chinese Medicine, disease is divided into excess conditions (yang) such as heat, pain, and hyper-function verses deficiency conditions (yin) such as weakness and hypo-function. In a subspecialty of oriental medicine, five-element acupuncture, it

---

[8] Pulse diagnosis of five element acupuncture: This is a primary tool used in acupuncture to access the health of the patient. It is based on the theory that the strength of the pulse on both radial arteries of the wrist vary along its path at the region of the styloid process. These variations relate to the organ meridian systems of the patient and the relative strength and weaknesses of each specific area can guide one to a treatment protocol. More about this later.

is believed that excesses are a result of an underlying deficiency as part of a negative feedback mechanism. When we treat the excess symptoms using conventional acupuncture, we do not cure the patient, we simple move the disease to another location (I term this translocation) in at least 90% of the patients. This "excessive pathological information", is mostly of an astral nature. These Yang structures are called luciferic demons.

- When we treat the deficiency after the control theory of five element acupuncture (see picture below), we also just translocate the "deficient pathological information" in about 40% of the patients, which is mostly of an etheric nature. These Yin structures are ahrimanic demons.
- If we treat the middle, which is the mid-point between excess (Yang or astral structure) and deficiency (Yin or etheric structure), we create the possibility of transforming the Luciferic structure and keeping the Ahrimanic demon at bay. This transformation then takes place in about 90% of the patients
- If we treat the middle when the patients are sitting in a group or a circle, it appears that we are able to address the spiritual foundations of the disease, but this method does not seem to have very good somatic changes.
- If we treat the middle from the already mentioned knowledge of the morning-evening forces as opposed to the midday-midnight forces, it seems that a combination of the anatomical middle point and the morning-evening-forces-point can transform close to 100% of the pathological structures residing in the body of the patients.

The 5-element star system of Chinese medicine is simply a negative feedback construct relating to the regulation between excess and deficiency and does not function well in finding and treating the middle point. Therefore, as a curative tool it has little validity and a new methodology must take its place.

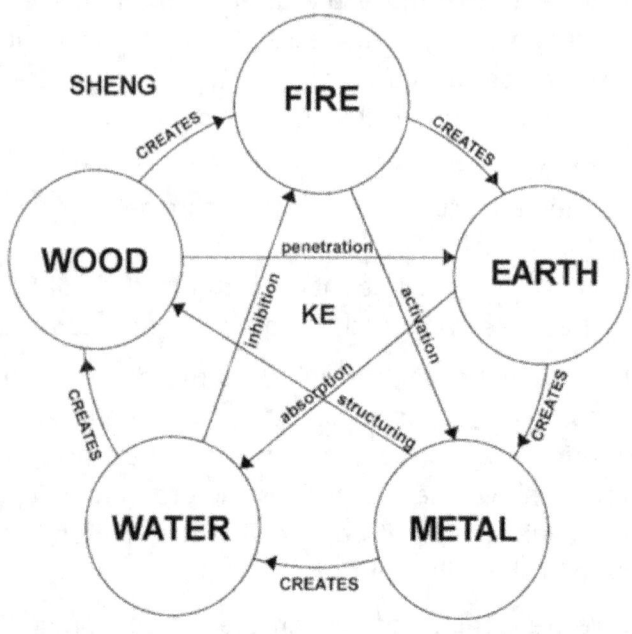

The Negative feedback model of the Five Elements

Leaving the thinking in 5-elements to thinking in 12-elements; The 12-element zodiacal system.

The zodiacal system as viewed as a quadratum (in a 90⁰ angel) (Order of processes as the constellations are ordered in the cosmos).

Where in this system:

- Gall-bladder heals Bladder (in a Christ/Sophia-like way).
- Liver heals Kidney (in a Christ/Sophia-like way).
- Spleen heals Large Intestine (in a Christ/Sophia-like way).
- Small Intestine heals hormonal system (in a Christ/Sophia-like way).
- Bladder heals Liver (in a Christ/Sophia-like way).
- Large Intestine heals Stomach (in a Christ/Sophia-like way).
- hormonal system heals Heart (in a Christ/Sophia-like way).
- Liver heals Kidney (in a Christ/Sophia-like way).
- Stomach heals Lung (in a Christ/Sophia-like way).
- Heart heals Pericardium (in a Christ/Sophia-like way).
- Kidney heals Gall bladder (in a Christ/Sophia-like way).
- Lung heals Spleen (in a Christ/Sophia-like way).

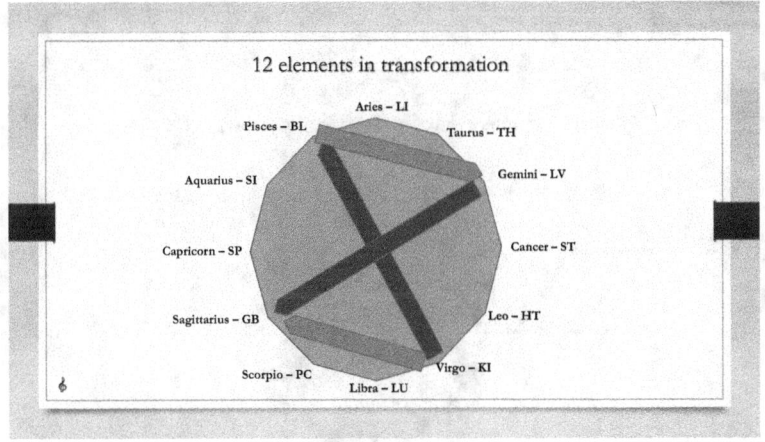

In this system we have 3 quadrats:

1. Hormonal system – Heart – Pericardium – Small Intestine.
   This is the feeling-inter(by love)-healing-system.
2. Liver – Kidney – Gall bladder – Bladder.
   This is the willing-inter(by love)-healing-system.
3. Stomach – Lung – Spleen – Large intestine.
   This is the thinking-inter(by love)-healing-system.

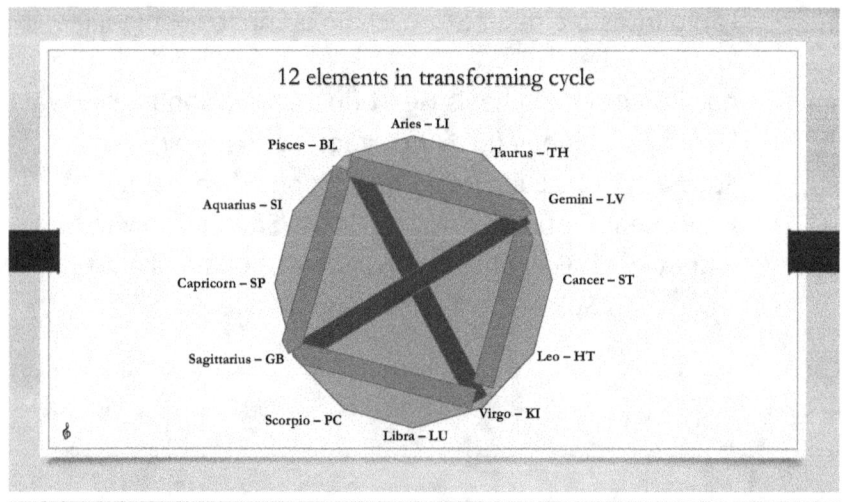

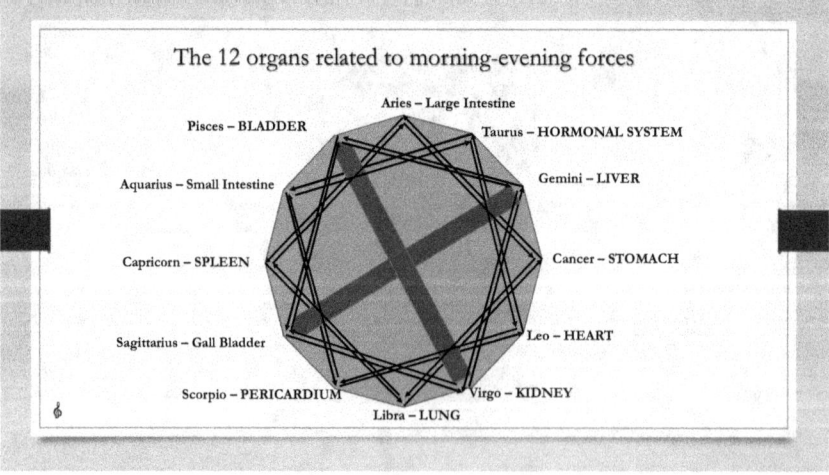

Where in this system:

- Liver and Gall-bladder heals Kidney and Bladder (in a Christ/Sophia-like way).
- Kidney and Bladder heals Liver and gall-bladder (in a Christ/Sophia-like way).
- Heart and Small Intestine heals Pericardium and Trippel Heather (in a Christ/Sophia-like way).
- Pericardium and Trippel Heather heals Heart and Small Intestine (in a Christ/Sophia-like way).
- Lung and Large Intestine heals Spleen and Stomach (in a Christ/Sophia-like way).
- Spleen and Stomach heals Lung and Large Intestine (in a Christ/Sophia-like way).

An explanation to the last figure.
Here, in this last figure we see how the masculine and feminine forces together can heal.

First, we had separated the masculine and the feminine from the 5-elemets to a 12 element-cycle, where the masculine and the feminine had been separated, and then, as shown in the last figure, both the masculine and the feminine can work together in healing the disease.

In this way liver and gall bladder can together heal both the kidney and the bladder.

In this way we will have:
1. Liver and Gallbladder together heals Kidney and Bladder and vica versa.
2. Lung and large Intestine together heals Spleen and Stomach and vica versa.

3. Heart and Small intestine together heals pericardium and Hormonal system and vica versa.

In this way man and woman, Christ and Sophia, join their forces in healing the world.

Salvatore Mundi.

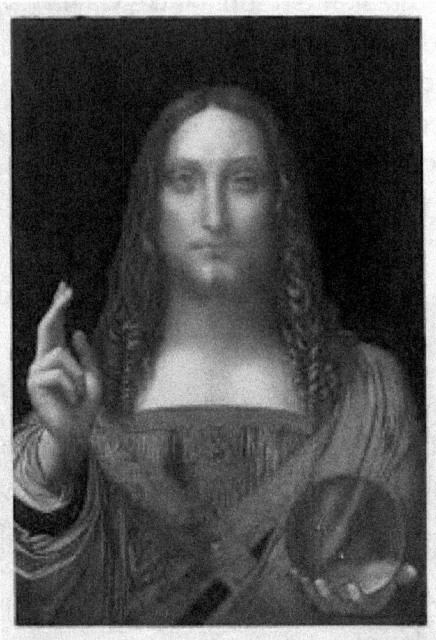

The only true path to cure is through Christ consciousness as described by the science of Anthroposophy. This is accomplished through the middle point, a point that relates to the Christ-consciousness. As I evolved in my understanding of this phenomenon, I found that there are actually three anatomical middle points located anatomically at a midpoint in each of three areas of the body. Furthermore, these regions relate to the soul faculties of thinking, feeling and willing. The importance of individualizing these functions will become apparent as you continue reading this book. Listed below are the locations of these three middle points:

- The middle point of the cranium, representing thinking
- The middle point of the sternum, representing feeling
- The middle point of the lower abdomen or lumbo-sacrum, representing willing

All middle points are found halfway between the excess as represented by the Luciferic structure, and the deficiency, the location of the Ahrimanic structure. Furthermore, the exact location of this middle point can be determined by developing a clairvoyant or spiritual equivalent of seeing, feeling, hearing, tasting or smelling. Keep in mind, we are using these "spiritual" senses to perceive the healthy area where the healing energy of Christ is located. For some, this is perceived, using a spiritual eye, as an area of white light. However, to gain the ability to perceive these spiritual visions requires the ability to enter into the spiritual world. These methods appear unorthodox but can be learned through the exercises found in anthroposophy and spiritual science.

To understand what I am about to share with the reader will change your reality regarding all medical treatment. Everything that is revealed in this book, the existence of demons, the transforming effect of the Christ-point, group therapy, and the meaning behind an anthroposophic wooden statue entitled the group, will no doubt challenge the belief system held by most of you. To move forward, to create a true model of healing, we must come to grips with a new reality which includes the fact that the middle point is not an acupuncture point, rather a sacred entry into the Christ consciousness lying between the two adversaries that cause so much suffering.

In the beginning of my practice I had observed that my consciousness about the life and existence of trees, of the life of nature in general, had a distinct effect on the results of my treatments. For example, I had been treating "Herpes Zoster" for some years, but had absolutely no results or effect on this disease. I then read a lecture of Rudolf Steiner about its spiritual causes, and immediately my clinical results changed from 0% to 90%, doing exactly the same treatment as I did before reading this lecture. I was amazed! It seems then, that the knowledge and understanding of diseases and how to treat them is of great importance to the outcome of the treatment. Now, with increasing frequency, the spiritual reality stretches its hands out into my life, inspiring the ideas to give birth to yet another new book.

One of my most important epiphanies occurred when I realized that diseases may be translocated after my "normal" alternative treatment. I had no idea how to avoid that. Later I learned and realized that in treating the middle or Christ point, either the anatomical point and/or the morning-evening-90^0-point, this effect might be avoided, especially concerning the luciferic demons, and to a lesser extent the ahrimanic ones.

Chapter 2:

The Three-fold way: Thinking, Feeling, Willing.

Many years ago, I started to "spiritually see" the pathological processes as demonic entities, gaining entrance into the body as a result of the weaknesses, faults and mistakes in living made by the patient. As mentioned previously, there are at least two kinds of such entities; the luciferic and the ahrimanic. The luciferic pathological entity is situated closer to the head (proximal), while the ahrimanic pathological entity is closer to the base of the spine (distal).

These demonic structures were once considered elemental beings, spiritual entities not considered malevolent. Just like bacteria, the presence of benign spiritual structures is both important and necessary to our human existence. It is when these forces created by Lucifer and Ahriman are mutated by weakness and faults in thinking, feeling and willing, that these entities become demonic and adversarial to health.

In 2012, I discovered the importance of treating the middle point, thinking and hoping that this should hinder the translocation.

In 2014, I started to realize, that my middle-point treatment still pushed the demonic entities outward only to either later return or to invade another host, although in a much lesser degree that when treating the excess or the deficiency. I still had to find methods to totally avoid translocation, and that there needed to be an attempt made to transform them with the intention of selfless love. When treating through the middle point it was somewhat possible to transform the luciferic entities, while the ahrimanic structures at this time, showed less evidence of transformation.[9]

In 2016, I discovered how the spiritual foundations could transform if the middle point was treated in a group, although the physical symptoms did not often change. Both the middle and its treatment with a group of patients will be discussed in the third section of this book.

In 2019 I discovered that the whole 5-element thinking was a deceit, even into the position of the pulses in pulse-diagnosis. I then changed the 5-elemetal thinking into a 12-elemental thinking and corrected the pulse-positions, and then I got even better results relating to transforming the pathological forces of disease.

I also realized that the wooden statue made by Rudolf Steiner and Edith Maryon, standing today in The Gotheanum, the center for Anthroposophy in Dornach, Switzerland, was actually a presentation of a cosmic spiritual treatment, where Christ is situated in the middle, separating Lucifer and Ahriman. During this separation, the face of the *"Cosmic Humour"* appears above the Christ figure. I studied in detail how the hands were held, how the fingers were pointed and how the handgrip between Lucifer and Ahriman was done. All this resembled in detail what I had observed in my treatment. I came to understand that this statue inhabited the solution to a totally spiritualized therapy.

In 2017, after a closer examination of "the group", I then discovered that there are two more middle-points between two Lucifers and two Ahrimans depicted in the group statue. I then realized that although there is a middle point located along the

---

[9] According to anthroposophy, Lucifer was once an angelic being, who through a serious misdeed, has been temporarily extracted from his lofty domain. Ahriman, however, descended to the depths of the lower world and was prevented access to the spirit world by its guardian, Archangel Michael. Thus, the difficulty for his demonic entities to be transformed.

sternum, there are also two more areas of potential treatment. The second location is found somewhere between the distal aspect of the sternum to the pubis. The third Middle point with its associated demons is located somewhere along the midline of the cranium. I have concluded that the cranium middle point is associated with the soul faculty of thinking, the sternal middle point with feeling, and the lower, abdominal middle point with willing. These points therefore can be selected based on the patient's particular pathology.

Note that the original middle point, located on the sternum, is the location for the two important chakras, the Heart chakra and the Throat chakra. It has been postulated in anthroposophic circles, that this is where the main attack of the adversarial forces will be launched.

This book is therefore written based on the foundation of the three soul faculties described by Rudolf Steiner.

1. The wooden statue of the "Group", demonstrating the Representative of Humanity (Christ) in all its details. This depicts the soul faculty of Love (Feeling).
2. The contents of Steiner's School of Spiritual Science summarizing how to enter the spirit world in a series of 19 + 7 lectures. This depicts the soul faculty of willing.
3. The enormous totality of anthroposophic philosophy according to Rudolf Steiner. This aspect represents the soul faculty of thinking.

It seems that the trinity of thinking, feeling and willing is the foundation of everything and everything can be under its construct. Examples of this include the three middle points, the three parts of the soul, the three adversarial forces of Lucifer, Ahriman and Azuras, the three divine forces of God, Christ and the Holy Spirit and so on.

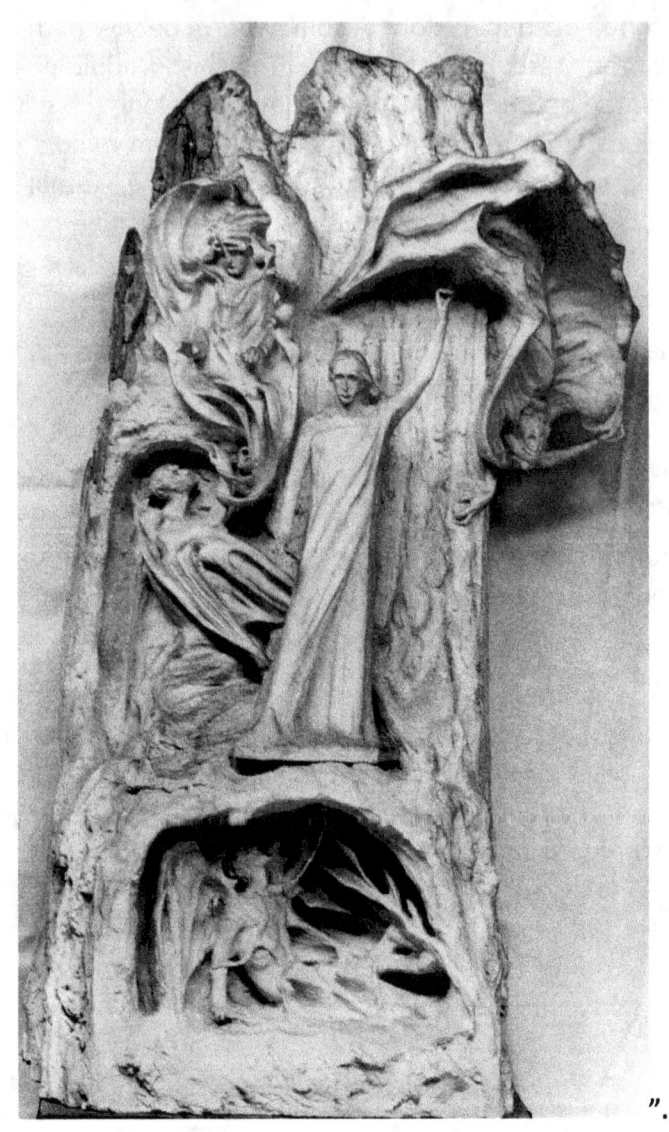

"The Group"

Chapter 3:

-Thinking, Feeling, and Willing in a Clinical Setting

As I will emphasize throughout this book, the ability to properly diagnose and successfully cure chronic disease requires the fundamental understanding and separate use of the soul faculties of *thinking*, *feeling* and *willing*: an important and fundamental aspect of Anthroposophy.

As a healer, the soul force of *thinking* involves the objective ability to gather data regarding diagnosis. Then, without prejudice, we must keep our *feelings* separated from our thoughts and refrain from performing a treatment (*willing*) until all the data is amassed. I have come to understand, through the teachings of Rudolf Steiner, that the only path into spiritual healing begins with training ourselves to separate these three soul faculties. And in opening this door, three new doors reveal themselves; one door through the pure thinking, one door through pure feeling and one door through pure willing. All these three doors must be opened to be able to enter the spiritual world properly. In fact, the entanglement of these qualities is what anchors us to the material and limits our ability to enter the supra sensory world. This entanglement creates the illusion that the only reality is contained in the physical universe. We believe that these soul faculties are produced within our physical brain rather than flowing into us from the spirit world. The true content, function, and power of these three soul forces are then overshadowed and hidden. It is the same as believing that the colors in the world are located in the eye and sounds come from the ear, created as well by the brain.

However, the real force of thinking, feeling and willing is not to the same extent hidden from us. The simplest force to separate is our ability to think, the most difficult is our ability to will. The soul faculty of feeling, however, lies somewhere in between our conscious and unconscious state.

Therefore, in order to be aware of their cosmic origin, and the immense forces that are hidden within thinking, feeling and willing, we have to separate them from each other. If thinking, feeling and willing are liberated, i.e. set free from one another, they can perform wonders. The reason for this is that in the separation of thinking, feeling and willing we become part of the cosmos, a part of God, and part of the Spiritual World.

The Separation of Thinking, Feeling and Willing (the southern way or stream).

Rudolf Steiner emphasized that the entanglement of Thinking, Feeling and Willing, the three cosmic forces originating in the spiritual world, is the main reason why we are anchored to the physical world. This is of crucial importance to the readers of this book, especially those desiring to connect with their higher self.

When man, consisting of body, soul and spirit, incarnates in the physical world, our Feeling, Thinking and Willing are entangled, intertwined, and bound together. The real content, function, and power of the three Soul Faculties, are hidden from us because they overshadow each other. Modern medicine would have us believe that Thinking, Feeling and Willing are just faculties developed or produced by ourselves, and forever interdependent. This is a serious mistake that keeps us in ignorance, otherwise known as Maya[10]. This is what Morpheus and Neo in the film *"The*

---

[10] **Maya** (Sanskrit: माया māyā) literally "illusion", "magic", has multiple meanings in Indian philosophies depending on the context. In ancient Vedic literature, māyā literally implies extraordinary power and wisdom. In later Vedic texts and modern literature dedicated to Indian traditions, māyā connotes a "magic show,

Matrix" experienced, depicting reality as a dream state induced by a computer program in order to control us as a species. It is what we might call the *"greater illusion"*[11].

It is as if we would believe that the colors are within the eye, created by ourselves, and that the sounds are within the ear, created by the brain. It is the same with Thinking, Feeling and Willing. These are three cosmic forces which we may use as our own, and as such become part of the cosmos, the divine, and the spirit world.

We can facilitate healing that often appears miraculous if we learn to separate, these 3 soul faculties in our diagnosis and treatment.

- Willing is the strongest but most hidden power.
- Feeling is the half-conscious and half-hidden power.
- Thinking is the least hidden power.

To be aware of the cosmic origin of the three soul faculties, and to use the immense forces hidden within them in clinical practice, we must learn, how to separate them. We can achieve this separation by knowing their secrets[12], but also through meditation and concentration. Other ways that these faculties separate are through sunstroke or fainting, neurological diseases such as

---

an illusion where things appear to be present but are not what they seem". Māyā is also a Spiritual concept connoting "that which exists but is constantly changing and thus is Spiritually unreal", and the "power or the principle that conceals the true character of Spiritual reality".

[11] **The greater and lesser illusion:** Although the greater illusion describes the illusion of the material world, the lesser illusion is within the Spiritual world itself, when souls abiding there are lost or stuck in the belief that there is no way out, no way to reincarnate, no love and no Christ.

[12] The knowledge of the true origin of Thinking, Feeling and Willing are described by many mystics and in many of the mysteries through the ages, among others by Rudolf Steiner in his Anthroposophy.

epilepsy, or by dying. As I mentioned in the introduction, for many years, although I never had "grand mal" convulsions, I thought that I suffered from epilepsy, as the symptoms resembled its description. I now realize that these symptoms represented a spontaneous separation of my Thinking, Feeling and Willing.

This separation often, if not always, opens one's being to a spiritual reality, something essential for our spiritual development. On his way to Damascus, Saint Paul (then called Saul) experienced these phenomena. In that awakening, he felt and saw the existence of Christ. St. Paul's Epistle to the Galatians [Galatians 1:11-16] describes his conversion as a divine revelation, in which Jesus Christ appeared to him:

> "I want you to know ... that the gospel I preached is not of human origin. I did not receive it from any man, nor was I taught it; rather, I received it by revelation from Jesus Christ. For you have heard of my previous way of life in Judaism, how intensely I persecuted the church of God and tried to destroy it ... But when God ... was pleased to reveal his Son in me so that I might preach him among the Gentiles, my immediate response was not to consult any human being".

However, many doctors attribute Paul's ecstatic vision and conversion to an epileptic seizure. For example, J Neurol Neurosurg Psychiatry, 1987, 50(6): 659–664 [PMC1032067] in a paper regarding this subject, states:

> "St Paul and temporal lobe epilepsy: Evidence is offered to suggest a neurological origin for Paul's ecstatic visions. Paul's physical state at the time of his conversion is discussed and related to these ecstatic experiences. It is postulated that both were manifestations of temporal lobe epilepsy".

Thus, just as they question the "Elf-School" and the "Angel-School", atheists question the story of St. Paul's spiritual awakening.

From my earliest childhood memories of the phenomenon, the symptoms of "spontaneous separation" of Thinking, Feeling and Willing started with my inability to judge distances. Depth ceased to have any meaning. The next loss I suffered was the ability to perceive width. In addition, height disappeared from my consciousness. I felt like I was floating in space without having the perception of a dimensional reality. Finally, the concept of time vanished. I had no immediate concept of how long these moments lasted, although I could see from my watch that they usually ended in less than an hour. In this way, I lost more and more of my physical reality, leading to the separation of my three soul faculties.

Through these experiences I discovered that Thinking is connected to height, Feeling is associated with an outward movement (width) and Willing (depth) is connected to the downward direction. In summary, by the end of my "fit", the concept of time and space became meaningless. This is similar to the description of the epileptic fit of the author, *Dostoevsky* in his book *"The Idiot"*.

Of course, as a young child, I was frightened by my excarnations. However, as I grew older, I began to enjoy entering the spirit world. Finally, in my 35th year, I decided to use acupuncture to cure myself of my condition. As soon as the next "fit" appeared, I inserted myself with a needle at the appropriate point and with the explosive sensation of a jet passing through my head, the spontaneous fits ceased, never to return.

However, the knowledge of how to separate depth, height, width and time remained. As a consequence, I retained the ability to separate Thinking, Feeling and Willing. I use this method successfully every time I want to observe energy patterns in patients, trauma within the body or to see the inhabitants of the spiritual world, such as elves, gnomes or even demons.

Because of this ability, I quit traditional veterinary work and began to employ acupuncture and a diagnostic technique of Traditional Chinese Medicine entitled pulse-diagnosis as my daily tool.

What is the "I"?

According to Spiritual Science, the human organization consists of a trinity of a body, soul and spirit. The physical human body is adapted to the conditions of the material world and has needs stemming from this fact. The spirit, however is directed to the freedom of the spiritual world. While the physical body is held captive to eating and drinking, the spirit has the freedom to make decisions regarding reading a book, painting a picture, meditating, and so on. The soul lies somewhere between the body and spirit, having characteristics of both. The soul has a sentient aspect (controlling the senses), an intellectual aspect (logical reasoning) and a conscious aspect (the concept of individuality). This latter aspect of the soul allows the individual free will to decide to re-enter the divine world or be tempted by evil.

The spirit is also referred to as the I, denoting our self and our associated ego. The I consciousness of man accounts for our uniqueness as a living being on this planet. It includes our memory, our speech, our erect posture and our ability to rationalize. This is especially important when given a choice that involves our conscious. The" I" is immortal returning once and again in new incarnations. This immortality relates more to the spiritual essence than our own ego. The "I" is responsible for the various impulses of the new life. This can lead to situations where we can repair harms done in past lives, as well as facilitate the progress of other people and humanity. These situations create a destiny that can involve meeting certain people, traveling to certain places, or even developing certain diseases. However, what we do with these synchronicities is our free choice.

The concept of the "I" is further divided into three separate members. Keep in mind, at this stage in our evolution, the I is far from evolved. The lowest I, called the spirit self, acts on the astral body. The next one, named the life spirit, acts on the ether body, and the third, the spirit person, constitutes the human individuality in the spirit world.

The Separation of the etheric body and the astral body (the northern way or stream).

Personal comments and description of The Nordic stream, a method I always use when taking the pulse-diagnosis.

Personally I always gone directly into the spiritual world when taking the pulse (or when seeing elemental beings or spirits or demons).

To do this we must divide the astral from the etheric, leading to also separating thinking, feeling and willing, as well as time itself, if we want to proceed further.

This method was first described by Steiner in 1910[13] (as far as I know), namely how to pass the 'Threshold' without encountering this 'Guardian' phenomenon, this reflection and awareness of one's own weaknesses in connection with the threshold crossing itself. This method involves retaining (in the morning, upon awakening), or introducing (through the day otherwise) a partial,

---

[13] Lecture held on the 24th of Mars 1910 (GA 119).

more or less, separation between the etheric body and the astral body.

I have described this in detail in my books ... "Demons - Healing" (published at Temple Lodge, 2018) "Experiences from the Threshold" (published at Temple Lodge, 2019) and "Translocation" (Amazon, 2019)

I have always perceived that there are three main avenues for spiritual enlightenment, three avenues offered in anthroposophy.

1. The 'Christian' way, focused study of John the Gospel (via the heart - the feeling - the door of the sun).
2. The "Rosen cross" path, which is essentially described in Steiner's "How to gain knowledge of the higher worlds" (via the head - thinking - the gate of death).
3. A way (the most modern and secure) based on working with both the content and the form of Steiner's 'philosophy of freedom' (via the limb system - the will - the door of the elements).

However, it has never been quite clear what exactly this last path entails (working with 'The Philosophy of Freedom') and how to ideally walk it, how it differs from the work one can do with other philosophical texts and what exercises it actually contains. By studying this book, we gain the opportunity to learn and practice the ability to connect observation with concepts, and how this insight is the basis for our freedom and the development of mindless thinking (pure thinking and will), and how this can help us to live a moral life, a life of 'ethical individualism'. But the study of this book does not seem to describe a specific path into the spiritual world.

To me, the description of the three paths looks like a variation of the description of:

- The door of death (thinking - meeting the third animal).
- The door of the elements (the will - meeting the first animal).
- The sun's door (the feeling - meeting the second animal).

One is through thinking, the other through emotion and the third through will.

The referred 'direct' path can be described as a possible fourth path[14], a kind of 'shortcut' into the spiritual world without immediately meeting the 'Guardian of the Threshold'.

Instead, this encounter is transformed into a lifelong encounter with Karma in the physical world.

This is a path that can be characterized as 'a middle path', a path between thinking and feeling, between feeling and will, or even between the astral and the etheric body.

This 'shortcut' is described by Rudolf Steiner in 1910 in Helsinki, in a lecture on 7/10-1904 in Berlin on "Prometheus"[15] (GA 92) (also referred to in the "Temple legend"[16] (GA 93)). Likewise in Chapter 5 of "Christianity as a Mysterious Fact" (GA 8), in "Pastoral Medicine" (GA 318), in a lecture held in Helsinki on April 3, 1912

---

[14] With the possible exception, the "Cognitive Yoga" method described by Isaiah Ben-Aharon can also be described as a "fourth way". In that case, the way described by me here is a "fifth way". On the other hand, Ben-Aharon's explanation of the first stages of 'cognitive yoga' begins by describing the electrolysis of water to two gases, hydrogen and oxygen, a scientific analogy that helps explain the process of separating and 'etherizing' perception and mental imagination. The goal is to experience a pure sense-perception and a pure thinking separately as free etheric forces. In this way, his "Cognitive Yoga Method" may be an example of the general path of division I describe in this article.

[15] Lecture held 7th of January 1904 (GA 92).

[16] Lecture on the 'Temple-legend', lecture 4, 1904 (GA 93).

(GA 136), and last but not least in the last two the lectures given in England in 1924 on 'True and False Paths in Spiritual Investigations', given in Torquay (GA 243).

In Parsifal and Kalevala, too, this method is described.

This method is, in my opinion, particularly suitable for the Nordic peoples, perhaps since Steiner described it in detail in Helsinki in 1912, that Parsifal experienced it on a winter's day in the snow and that it is described in the only song in Kalevala that can relate to the existence of Christ, namely in the 50th song that tells of Marjatta.

I will now further describe this possible fourth way in a personal way, a road described by Rudolf Steiner as a kind of "shortcut" into the spiritual world without immediately meeting the "Guardian of the Threshold". This meeting is instead transformed into a lifelong meeting with Karma in the physical world[17].

This is a path that can be characterized as "a middle way", a path *between* thought and feeling, *between* feeling and will or even *between* the astral and the etheric body.

This is described by Rudolf Steiner in 'Pastoral Medicine'[18]:

> *"Let us consider first what the situation is when the astral body and ego approach the etheric body. In clairvoyance*

---

[17] It is thus, in my opinion, different levels of clairvoyance, apart from the descriptions Steiner made of imaginative, inspirative and intuitive clairvoyance, and these levels may be characterized by the path chosen; the astral path (the usual path), the etheric path (the direct path), the physical path (probably through the resurrection body) and possibly a spiritual path (used by the initiates).

[18] 'Pastoral Medicine', Lecture 8, 15. September 1924 (GA 318).

one can bring this condition about fairly easily, by strengthening thinking - strengthening it by very thorough, energetic meditation. Then it is easy to come to this condition; it is the beginning of initiation. One slips down into the etheric body but is not yet able to take hold of the physical body; one remains in the etheric body. In this condition it is possible to think very, very well. One sees nothing, hears nothing, but one can think very well. Thinking is not in the least extinguished, but seeing, hearing and the other sense activities are suppressed. At first, thinking remains the same, except that one can think more than previously. One can think such thoughts as we are expressing here, for instance thought about the macrocosm. Thinking becomes wider. One knows clearly; 'now I am in the etheric world.' Thus, when one is in the etheric body, one is truly in the world ether. One has the clear experience of this: 'I am in the spiritual world out of which the sense world comes.' But one is not able to differentiate between spiritual world and sense world, one is beyond a differentiated sense world. The sun no longer shines, the stars no longer shine, there is no moonlight. There is no longer a clear distinction between the kingdoms of nature on the earth. A person only has that faculty when down in the physical body in normal life or in a higher stage of initiation. But in exchange for the blurring of the contours of the sense world., there is a general spirituality, the weaving life of the spirit.

In going this 'direct' way, one must then perform twelve important works (through all the zodiacal realities or also relating to all the twelve sensory organs) in the physical world (or at the intersection of the physical and the etheric world), so that through the suffering experienced in these twelve tasks or works, one comes to the knowledge of the Zodiac.

One will then learn to know the macrocosm and microcosm, which is hinted at in the lecture held on August 21, 1924, Torquay, in England (GA 243).

Instead of meeting the 'Guardian' on or directly behind the Threshold to the spiritual world, we than have to perform 12 important deeds in the physical world, or in the crossing between the physical and the spiritual worlds, so that one through effort and pain will arrive at knowledge about the astral forces of the universe, the Zodiac.

These 12 'Hercules'-deeds are related to the 12 steams related to the forces streaming in from the universe, the cosmic etheric forces. These forces materialize in the 12 organs that make us able to express ourselves in the material world.

In this way we again find a relation or connection to the therapy through the middle, the 900-morning-evening-forces and the 12-elemental zodiac.

Hercules 12 deeds

In a fit of madness, induced by Hera, Heracles killed his children and Megara. After his madness had been cured with hellebore by Antikyreus, the founder of Antikyra, he realized what he had done and fled to the Oracle of Delphi. Unbeknownst to him, the Oracle was guided by Hera. He was directed to serve King Eurystheus for ten years and perform any task Eurystheus required of him. Eurystheus decided to give Heracles ten labors, but after completing them, Heracles was cheated by Eurystheus when he added two more, resulting in the Twelve Labors of Heracles.

The labors of Hercules are not recounted in any single place, but must be reassembled from many sources. Ruck and Staples assert that there is no one way to interpret the labors, but that six were located in the Peloponnese, culminating with the rededication of Olympia. Six others took the hero farther afield, to places that were, per Ruck, "all previously strongholds of Hera or the 'Goddess' and were Entrances to the Netherworld". In each case, the pattern was the same: Hercules was sent to kill or subdue, or to fetch back for Eurystheus (as Hera's representative) a magical animal or plant.

A famous depiction of the labors in Greek sculpture is found on the metopes of the Temple of Zeus at Olympia, which date to the 450s BC.

In his labors, Hercules was sometimes accompanied by a male companion (an *eromenos*), according to Licymnius and others, such as Lolaus, his nephew. Although he was supposed to perform only ten labors, this assistance led to two labors being disqualified: Eurystheus refused to recognize slaying the Hydra, because Lolaus helped him, and the cleansing of the Augean stables, because Hercules was paid for his services and because the rivers did the work. Several of the labors involved the offspring (by various accounts) of Typhon and his mate Echidna, all overcome by Hercules.

A traditional order of the labors found in the *Bibliotheca*[19] is:

1. Slay the Nemean lion (deed of the Heart or the Lion).
2. Slay the nine-headed Lernaean Hydra (deed of the Stomach or the **Cancer**).
3. Capture the Ceryneian Hind (deed of the Blood circulation (Pericardium) or the **Scorpio**).
4. Capture the Erymanthian Boar (deed of the Lungs or the **Libra**).
5. Clean the Augean stables in a single day (deed of the Small Intestine or the **Aquarius**).

---

[19] Pseudo-Apollodorus: *Bibliotheke* 2.5.1-2.5.12.

6. Slay the Stymphalian birds (deed of the Gall bladder or the **Sagittarius**).
7. Capture the Cretan Bull (deed of the Hormonal system or the **Taurus**).
8. Steal the Mares of Diomedes (deed of the Large intestine or the **Aries**).
9. Obtain the girdle of Hippolyta (deed of the Kidneys or the **Virgo**).
10. Obtain the cattle of the monster Geryon (deed of the Urinary bladder or the **Pisces**).
11. Steal the apples of the Hesperides (deed of the Liver or the Gemini).
12. Capture and bring back Cerberus (deed of the Spleen or the **Capricorn**)[20].

One will then get to know the macrocosm and the microcosm.

This 'technique' is described by Steiner in a lecture held in Finland[21], where he says as follows:

> *Suppose a human soul gazes in this way at nothing but the blue of the sky. A certain moment then comes, a moment in which the blue-sky ceases to be blue — in which we no longer see anything which can in human language be called blue. If at that moment when the blue to us ceases to be blue, we turn our attention to our own soul, we shall notice quite a special mood in it. The blue disappears, and*

---

[20] The relations between the deeds and the Zodiacal signs are taken from the works of Kristin O´Donnell Tubb, and the relations to the organs are taken from my own clinical experiences as a therapist.

[21] Lecture held in Helsinki on the 3de of April 1912 (GA 136).

as it were, an infinity arises before us, and in this infinity a quite definite mood in our soul; a quite definite feeling, a quite definite perception pours itself into the emptiness which arises where the blue had been before. If we would give a name to this soul perception, to that which would soar out there into infinite distances, there is only one word for it; it is a devout feeling in our soul, a feeling of pious devotion to infinity. All the religious feelings in the evolution of humanity have fundamentally a nuance which contains within it what I have here called a pious devotion; the impression of the blue vault of the heavens which stretches above us has called up a religious feeling, a moral perception. When within our souls the blue has disappeared, a moral perception of the external world springs to life.

Let us now reflect upon another feeling by means of which we can in another way attune ourselves in moral harmony with external nature. When the trees are bursting into leaf and the meadows are filled with green, let us fix our gaze upon the green which in the most varied manner covers the earth or meets us in the trees; and again we will do this in such a way as to forget all the external impressions which can affect our souls, and simply devote ourselves to that which in external nature meets us as green. If once more we are so circumstanced that we can yield ourselves to that which springs forth as the reality of green, we can carry this so far that the green disappears for us, in the same way as previously the blue as blue disappeared. Here again we cannot say, "a color is spread out before our sight," but (and I remark expressly that I am telling you of things that everyone can experience for himself if he fulfils the requisite conditions) the soul has instead a peculiar feeling, which can be thus expressed: "I now understand what I experience when I think creatively, when a thought springs up in me, when an idea strikes me: I understand this now for the first time, I can only learn this from the bursting forth of the green all around me. I begin to understand the inmost parts of my soul through external nature when the outer natural impression has disappeared and, in its place, a moral impression is left. The green of the plant tells me how I ought to feel within myself, when my soul is blessed with the power to think thoughts, to cherish ideas."

Here again an external impression of nature is transmuted into a moral feeling.

Or again we may look at a wide stretch of white snow. In the same way as in the description just given of the blue of the sky and the green of earth's robe of vegetation, so this too can set free within us a moral feeling for all that we call the phenomenon of matter in the world. And if, in contemplation of the white snow mantle, we can forget everything else, and experience the whiteness, and then allow it to disappear, we obtain an understanding of that which fills the earth as substance, as matter. We then feel matter living and weaving in the world. And just as one can transform all external sight-impressions into moral perceptions, so too can one transform impressions of sound into moral perceptions. Suppose we listen to a tone and then to its octave, and so attune our souls to this dual sound of a tonic note and its octave that we forget all the rest, eliminate all the rest and completely yield ourselves to these tones, it comes about at last that, instead of hearing these dual tones, our attention is directed from these and we no longer hear them. Then again, we find that in our soul a moral feeling is set free. We begin then to have a spiritual understanding of what we experience when a wish lives within us that tries to lead us to *something, and then our reason influences our wish. The concord of wish and reason, of thought and desire, as they live in the human soul, is perceived in the tone and its octave.*

What is described here is like the technique I use to separate the ethereal and the astral.

If we then make this mental division into our spiritual make-up, the etheric world will manifest itself to us, as further described by Steiner[22]:

In like manner we might let the most varied sense perceptions work upon us; we could in this way let all that we perceive in nature through our senses disappear, as it were, so that this sense-veil is removed; then moral perceptions of sympathy and antipathy would arise everywhere. If we accustom ourselves in this way to eliminate all that we see with our eyes, or hear with our

---

[22] I will at this point in my description make a remark on the differences between an astral, an etheric, a physical and a spiritual clairvoyance. In reaching or developing an astral clairvoyance first the seer is prone to observe his own astral projections, and may very well be mistaken in his observations. This is not so great danger in the etheric clairvoyance, as it is much more difficult to manipulate the etheric world than it is the astral world. In a physical clairvoyance the phantom or resurrection body is used, and this is almost impossible to manipulate. In a spiritual clairvoyance the total spiritual world relieves itself for the seer, and any manipulation is extremely seldom. This differentiation of the different clairvoyances is in my opinion not the same as the differentiation between an imaginative, an inspirative and an intuitive consciousness, as all these three may be applied within all the four kinds of clairvoyances, a total of 12 possibilities.

ears, or that our hands grasp, or that our understanding (which is connected with the brain) comprehends — if we eliminate all that, and accustom ourselves, nevertheless, to stand before the world, then there works within us something deeper than the power of vision of our eyes, or the power of hearing with our ears, or the intellectual power of our brain-thinking; we then confront a deeper being of the external world. Then the immensity of Infinity so works upon us that we become imbued with a religious mood. Then does the green mantle of plants so work upon us that we feel and perceive in our inner being something spiritually bursting forth into bloom. Then does the white robe of snow so work upon us that by it we gain an understanding of what matter, of what substance is in the world; we grasp the world through something deeper within us than we had hitherto brought into play. And therefore in this way we come into touch with something deeper in the world itself. Then, as it were, the external veil of nature is drawn aside, and we enter a world which lies behind this external veil. Just as when we look behind the physical body of man we come to the etheric or life-body, so in this way we come into a region in which, gradually, manifold beings disclose themselves — those beings which live and work behind the mineral kingdom, the plant kingdom, and the animal kingdom. The etheric world gradually appears before us, differentiated in its details.

By then entering the spiritual world by means of the described 'separation technique', by separating or translocating one of our spiritual 'constituents', the meeting(s) with the "Guardian of the Threshold" and 'his' reflection and awareness raised from our weaknesses will be shifted to the **material world**.

This is also described in my opinion with all the necessary clarity in **Wolfram von Eschenbach's** "Parsifal", written down at the end of the 12th century. This masterpiece of 24,810 verse lines describes Parsifal's path to "Gralen", that is, his initiation. At one point, in the sixth song, a profound transformation is described in Parsifal's soul. He sees three drops of blood in the white snow. He totally disappears "into" these drops, and his feelings separate from the rest of his soul. Then he meets, in the physical world, three opponents who challenge him and with whom he must fight. The three challengers are like the three animals Steiner describes in the meeting on the threshold, only that Parsifal must meet them in the physical wood. Having defeated the three contenders, described as thought, emotion and will, Parsifal is penetrated into the etheric world and can continue its quest for the Grail.

A further description by Rudolf Steiner we also find in lecture VII of "Man in the Light of Occultism" in Christiania (Oslo) on the 10th of June 1912 (GA 137):

> «When the occultist succeeds in experiencing in this way something like an after-image in respect of the human form — when, that is to say, having first comprehended this human form as he finds it in the physical world, he allows it then to "echo on" in him in the way that an after-image echoes on — when he is able to have this experience and afterwards to wait until the image of the human form is past and gone, he will obtain a picture of the human form which is no longer an image of the physical form but is experienced in the ether body.
>
> You see, for the pupil in occultism it is a question of experiencing himself in the ether body. And when the pupil has come to the point of experiencing himself in this way in the ether body, then this experience is indeed a profound one! It falls at once into two distinct experiences. It does not remain whole and single. And these two

> *experiences have to be expressed by two words. We have to say that the pupil experiences first, death and second, Lucifer.»*

Finally, in this article I would also like to relate what I have said here to the last two lectures Rudolf Steiner held in Torquay, in England[23], describing an initiation path that can be found at the intersection of sleep and awake, where the etheric and the astral are on the way to divorce or on the way to reunification.

In the, he says the following:

> *"We know, therefore, that by inner effort man brings the night consciousness into the day consciousness. When this happens in full consciousness, just as other activities are performed consciously during the day, when this vigilant man is able to invoke the night activities of the Moon into the waking experiences of the daytime, then he is on the true path. If he allows anything to enter into him when he is not fully conscious so that out of their own inner momentum the night experiences arise in the day consciousness, then he finds himself on the false path that ultimately leads to mediumism."*

Steiner emphasizes in these lectures that in this state the powers of the sun and the moon will work together, in some way intermingled. Steiner describes how the sun's forces work from within at night and from outside during the day, while the moon's powers work from the outside during the day and from within at night. A kind of reversal, which can often be seen as a

---

[23] lecture held on August 21, 1924, Torquay, in England (GA 243).

contradiction between the physical world and the etheric world, all is reversed.

Since I was three years old, I have experienced and worked on this technique, I wrote this poem as a 15-year-old boy about an experience I had when I was about 7 years of age, which quite accurately describes this "Threshold-experience" at the etheric initiation path.

The Angel

The doors are closed.

In one of the doors there is a little window,
and the handle is low enough
to be reached for the one that is small.

The door is open and the new spring-air flows in.

Not far away is the cherry-tree filled with its smell
and white flowers as the full, white moon.

I am new washed and it is Saturday.

Close to the cherry-tree trunk
a being is standing in the moonlight.

And even if it is day,
and all the others are sleeping their afternoon nap,
the entity is glowing in the dark.

Spiritual medicine, diagnosis, therapy and understanding as a pathway to initiation

Before I continue the discussion on the path to our higher self, I would like to quote Rudolf Steiner on this subject:

> "Between birth and death, man, at his present evolutionary stage, lives in ordinary life through three soul states: waking, sleeping, and the state between them, dreaming. Man acquires knowledge of higher worlds if he develops consciousness during sleeping. During its waking state the soul surrenders itself to sense-impressions and thoughts that are aroused by these impressions. During sleep the sense-impressions cease, but the soul also loses its consciousness. The experiences of the day sink into the sea of unconsciousness. Let us now imagine that the soul might be able during sleep to become conscious despite the exclusion of all sense-impressions. An answer to this problem is only possible if the soul is able to experience something even though no sense-activities and no memory of them are present in it. The soul, in regard to the ordinary outer world, would then find itself in a state similar to sleep, and yet it would not be asleep, but, as in the waking state, it would confront a real world. Such a state of consciousness can be induced if the human being can bring about the soul experiences made possible by spiritual science; and everything that this science describes concerning the worlds that lie beyond the senses.
>
> This state of consciousness resembles sleep only in a certain respect, namely, through the fact that all outer sense-activities cease with its appearance; also, all thoughts are stilled that have been aroused through these sense-activities. Through it a perceptive faculty is

awakened in the soul that in ordinary life is only aroused by the activities of the senses. The soul's awakening to such a higher state of consciousness may be called **initiation.**

The means of initiation lead from the ordinary state of waking consciousness into a soul activity, through which spiritual organs of observation are employed. These organs are present in the soul only in a germinal state; and must be developed. It may happen that a human being at a certain moment in the course of his life, without special preparation, makes the discovery in his soul that such higher organs have developed in him. This has come about as a sort of involuntary self-awakening. Such a human being will find that through it his entire nature is transformed. A boundless enrichment of his soul experiences occurs. He will find that there is no knowledge of the sense world that gives him such bliss, such soul satisfaction, and such inner warmth as he now experiences through the revelation of knowledge inaccessible to the physical eye. Strength and certainty of life will pour into his will from a spiritual world. There are such cases of self-initiation. They should, however, not tempt us to believe that this is the one and only way, and that we should wait for such self-initiation, doing nothing to bring about initiation through proper training.

The 7 recapitulation lessons from the School of Spiritual Science (based on the southern stream/way of initiation)

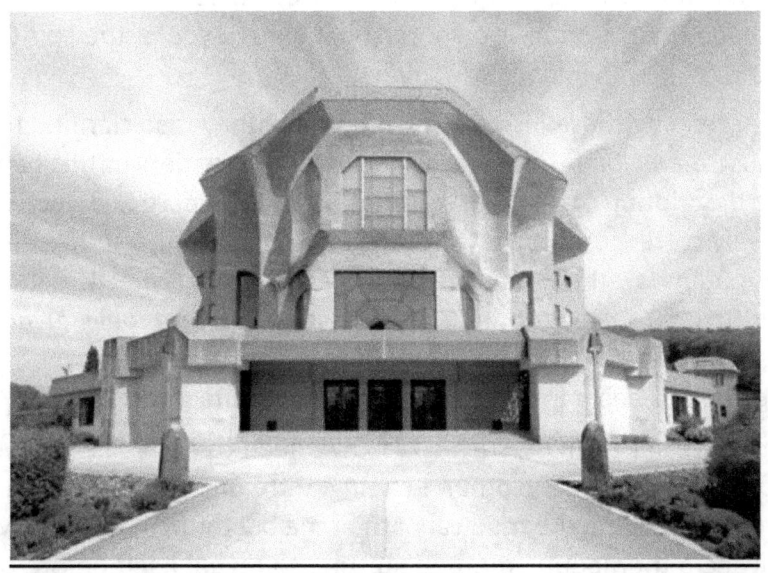

The Goetheanum, Dornach, Switzerland

After much political turmoil and decisiveness in the world of Anthroposophy, Rudolf Steiner re-founded the School for Spiritual Science in 1923. He dubbed this school "The Michael School"[24] after the archangel of the same name. He held these special lectures at the Goetheanum, in Dornach, Switzerland, his crowning architectural achievement that still stands as a mecca for anthroposophists around the world yearning for knowledge. Steiner was only able to give the first of three classes before his

---

[24] "Der Meditastionsweg der Michaelschule in neunzehn Stufen" Perseus Verlag, Basel, ISBN 978-3-907564-79-0

death. This class was comprised of nineteen original lessons followed by seven lessons which represented an elegant summary of the previous nineteen. He entitled the latter the "Seven Recapitulation Lessons". It was actually Rudolf Steiner's wish that we did not just quote these lessons but internalize them and reshape them from our own personal experience of the spiritual world.

After reading these lessons, my medical path was so clarified that I must share some of these insights with the readers of this book. The description of the path of initiation in these particular lectures closely corresponds to my lifelong attempt to immerse myself in my patient's etheric and astral forces by using what I feel is a spiritual pulse diagnosis. These lessons can not only give us assurance that we are on the right path, but also offer beneficial suggestions and corrections to help us expedite our journey

When we set forth on such a task, we need to read all the seven lectures, one after the other, in a single stream, with the intention of understanding the medical path of the doctor in mind. Then we will see a therapeutic method starting to reveal itself before our eyes.

1. The first lesson

In this lesson, the material world is described in all its glory, however, void of the true meaning of our existence and to why we are sick. The spiritual foundation of disease must be found elsewhere. Here we find the first and most fundamental command, without which we can't proceed. We must keep our heart open. We must also feel the longing for the spirit, together with the adoration of the creation. Then, with an open heart, we must pass the abyss to the spiritual world, to find the true cause of the disease. Before this is possible we have to divide our Thinking, Feeling and Willing.

We do this by sending our gaze out into the distance. This is also the first thing I do when I am about to examine a patient. I have to let my soul, my consciousness, and my gaze, fade out into the distant areas of the cosmos. By doing this, I start the separation of my feeling (which is in the distance) from the thinking (which is above) and my willing (which is below). To pass the abyss and enter the spirit world, we need to acquaint ourselves with these three forces of our soul; the thinking, the feeling and the willing. To do so, we must separate them to a certain extent. I do this when I approach a patient. I try to become totally aware of these three soul forces, and how I can differentiate them from one another, both in myself as well as in the patient.

Already, 30 years ago, I felt a darkness around me when I did this, and this is also described in the first lesson. We approach a dark, night-like wall, and this wall is the beginning of a deep darkness, the spiritual world, into which we are about to enter. In this darkness, we can and must hear with the heart, and this hearing with the heart is the only door (at least the most important and the first to be trodden. There are also two other doors to be opened, the door of the thinking and the door of the willing). Just behind the darkness, in front of the abyss that separates us from the spiritual world, we meet the Guardian of the threshold, and he makes us aware of the difficulties we may meet while we separate the three soul forces. In our thinking, we meet the doubt which must be met with hope, hatred, which must be met by love. In our feeling we meet the hatred, which must be met with love, and in our willing we meet the fear, which must be met by courage.

2. The second lesson

This lesson describes how we must be aware of the faults, wrongs, and shortcomings in our feelings, thoughts and will. This, according the Rudolf Steiner is visualized as the three frightening creatures that Fleming discussed in the previous chapter entitled the "Guardian of the threshold and the three animals".

As stated earlier, the guardian of the threshold to the spiritual world is there to both protect us and the spiritual world from us. These beasts are manufactured from our own mind showing us in vivid detail all the pain and harm we have reeked across space and time throughout our lives. We truly are awoken to the illusion of our false self. Thus, the beast of willing appears to show us our fear of manifesting true knowledge which can only be overcome by a having the courage to employ spiritual science in our daily life. The beast of feeling is born from our hatred of spiritual knowledge and can only be overcome by selfless love for all. And the beast of thinking can only be overcome if knowledge awakens in itself strength to create in one's own soul the things of the spiritual world beyond.

When the guardian shows us the shattering picture of our own being, we must realize that our previous thinking is no more than a dead corpse. We need to then realize that the way we feel things consumes and kills something in us. Without pure feeling, we are spiritually empty and must replace it with the true feeling of universal love. Then finally there is a falsehood of a will that is continually tempted by subversive forces who want to completely entangle us in earthly existence[25].

3. The third lesson

In this lesson, the guardian now shows us the path forward which leads to an ennoblement of self-knowledge. He explains that we should integrate ourselves into the cosmos, into the world with all its forces if we want to advance in our spiritual evolution. We do not obtain true knowledge if we remain in "our own skin". We must let our body become part of the entire world.

We are then told about the directions of the three soul powers. The thinking is up or above, the feeling is towards the far reaches

---

[25] As a personal comment, it is my experience that the appearance of the three animals is of a more benign nature than what Steiner experienced.

of the surroundings and the will is beneath in the direction of the center of the earth.

We consciously fade into the surroundings, leaving the thoughts and will behind, delving into the feeling. Then the physical world gets darker, we are unable to think and our will is gone, we are totally in the feeling. In this state, we are free from the laws of the physical world and can travel outside our body. In this state, we feel the warmth of the feeling, the light of the thinking and the life of the willing, as further described in the third lesson.

The first time I returned from the spiritual world, I experienced the utmost despair upon being presented with the fact that that my thoughts were dead and dark, my feelings were dead and cold and my will was weak and powerless. With this first-time experience in the back of my head, this option (death of the soul) is always present, always a possibility, and I see the animals each time I diagnose in this way

4. The fourth lesson

The pushing with the will deep into the spiritual layers of heart is described in the fourth lesson. The will has to enter the feeling, and together they must push. I then enter a sacred room, where I am in the etheric of the patient. At this point, I must activate the tip of my fingers, and they must press against the body of the patient, especially at a blood vessel. Often, I use the radial artery, but any place may be used. It is at this point that a total link is created, a connection between my feeling heart, my etheric fingers and my willing thinking. Using this link, I can begin my diagnostic work. I have to consider the disease of the patient and how it can be understood from a trinity.

When I am inside the etheric field of the patient, the following diagnostic questions arise: shall I consider him/her in relation to the 4 or the 5 elements? What about employing the 7 planets that are revealed in the bodily organs? Or perhaps I should consider or evaluate the patient in relation to the number 12? This can be in consideration of the 12 Zodiac Signs, the 12 meridians or the 12 fundamental processes of acupuncture. Every one of these possibilities are revealed in the 12 depths or layers of the body. (see next chapter for further explanation)

5. The fifth lesson

In this lesson, we are lectured about the necessity to allow our Will to enter the Thinking, and the Thinking to enter the Will. If will does not enter the thinking, pure cosmic thinking will overtake us, and we will be unable to think from our own "I". Furthermore, if the thinking does not enter the will, the cosmic Will overtakes us, and our Will becomes unusable. This happens also in the therapeutic process, where I let the Will and the Thinking mingle with each other, but always staying connected with the heart. It is as if the powers of the heart stream outwards, and in this process, attracts the Will and the Thinking. As such, the three soul forces then become one, and we are able to leave the diagnosis to begin therapy.

6. The sixth lesson

The sixth lesson describes further, how important it is, that the thinking is supported and connected to the Will. The thoughts must be willed in an outward movement, out into the world. The Will should also be infused with the Thinking, or else it will only work on its own. This fusing of Will and Thought *must* appear at the end of the diagnosis where we enter the stage of the therapeutic work; the impulse of the diagnosis must ascend into the therapy, into the world´s creative reality. The Feeling must be met by its own reality, by Feeling itself. In the spiritual world we, as a free spirit, first meet the patient in such a way that our Thinking, Feeling and Willing are more or less separated, then we meet them again as a diagnostician and lastly as a therapist. In this lesson, we actually cross the threshold, and it is at this juncture that we fundamentally change.

7. The seventh lesson: the phenomena of turning around

In the seventh lesson, the most important aspect of crossing the threshold is the act of turning around and looking back at the human part of ourselves, as we exist in the physical world. This is precisely what I must do as a therapist, when I want to finalize the therapeutic process. The patient, human or animal, is, in the first six lessons, taken apart as am I. We analyze, diagnose, treat, and heal both the patient and ourselves, and then everything is put back together again. We return to the physical world, back into the material reality. In this way, we now finish the journey into our therapeutic world. Before we go back into the physical universe, we must finalize this work. We now see the animals of the Abyss as the luciferic and ahrimanic demons, and we are able to place Christ right in the middle of them. The activation of Christ in the middle between Lucifer and Ahriman creates a balancing principle, and the symptoms and causes, as well as the excesses and deficiencies are dissipated. If we are to address the cooperation of Lucifer and Ahriman as an exacerbation of disease in the body, we first have to refrain from looking directly at them before turning around to face them. If we approach them directly, they are more easily translocated, driven to other parts of the body or even to other entities, humans or animals.

This is the deep mystery of "the turning around" which, when done correctly, will balance out the deficiencies as the transformed pathological structures disappear.

Conclusion regarding Thinking, Feeling and Willing

When the soul faculties are separated, we can then see Thinking as light and Will as a dark fire. Between the Thinking light and the fiery Will, the Feeling appears. All becomes *cosmic*. Karma and heritage works within our Will while Thoughts appear simultaneously in our head and at the same time in the Cosmos.

In other words, we will the thoughts so that they become cosmic. We let our feelings flow outward to thinking and willing so that the feeling becomes glorious. Finally, we must think our will and then the will becomes a force for a higher moral purpose.

SEE THE THREE.

Experience the world construction of the head.

Feel the world beating of the heart.

Think the power of the world in the limbs

A summary of some personal experiences with the 7 lessons

1. Regarding Time and the Spiritual world:

Rudolf Steiner describes, in the beginning of the 7 lessons, of how we can live in both the spiritual world and the physical world. However, he also warns us that we need to acknowledge that there are different laws relating to these two worlds. A good example of this relates to the concept of time

In pulse diagnosis, I go from a time frame of the material world (referred to as causality), which is actually an illusionary time, to the actual spiritual time, the time that is endless (continuum). In the Spiritual world, time simply *is*. I consider the latter an authentic concept that was corrupted by materialism. Material time destroys the power of real spiritual thinking. In other words, when entering the spiritual world, we go from cause and effect to a continuum, and then to an understanding. As described in the first and the second lesson concerning thinking: from the dead, to living and then a step further, to understanding.

2. Regarding The beasts of the abyss

When the animals of the abyss are described, I see them as a phenomenon. I see that part of the experience of crossing over is to transform these beasts. Then I am able to experience the living of real thinking (red), real feeling (yellow) and real willing (blue). I also have realized that the dangers in living in the spiritual world is the possibility of losing ourselves. This can be counteracted if we are able to obtain the balance in Christ. So, in a way, the first lesson describes the animals, the second what they are, and the third, how they may be conquered.

3. Regarding The directions of feeling, willing, and thinking

At the last part of the third lesson, the directions of the feeling, willing and thinking are described (will is downward, thinking upward, and feeling is outward to the surroundings), and the danger in going too far toward these directions. These vectors are important to understand and to be aware of as they also show themselves as the nine stages that I see when treating a Group (described in the third part of this trilogy). When a group or circle of people sit together, and the Christ force is activated in their Middle-Points, the healing-forces are first directed upwards, then downwards and then lastly outwards. In such a way, we may experience that in a real and true transformational healing, both the thinking, the willing and the feeling are healed, transformed and restored.

Additionally, the three forces of the soul, when separated, can alter the concept of gravity. This can be disorienting and I found that courage and love are necessary and important attributes that protect me from disorientation. Thus, the third lesson explains how darkness may overwhelm thinking, coldness may overwhelm feeling, and the fear of death, may overwhelm willing, ultimately creating a potential to drift too far into the three directions.

4. Regarding balancing as an important aspect of the spiritual world

When I direct my diagnosis and treatment toward creating a balance between Lucifer and Ahriman, I see that it is in this way the middle point can create healing through the Christ impulse. This balance is also visualized as a balance between warmth and cold. This was explained by Steiner in lesson 4.

When I master this balance, I can start to understand how to utilize the various numerical treatment protocols to best help the patient. These options are varied. I can apply the balance of the 4 elements (fire, earth, air, water), features of the 7 planets of Steiner (ie: Jupiter represents the function of the liver), or the 12 zodiac signs (ie: The meridian system of AP).

5. Regarding the aspect of touch

At this point of experiencing the spiritual world, touch is of special importance as it is the central part of pulse-diagnosis[26]. The touch of the fingers pressing on the blood coursing through the radial artery represents the fusion of willing and feeling. As healers, this is the understanding we are searching for. The Body is the element of earth, touch is water, life is air and feeling is fire. I can, in this way visualize myself in the elements. I feel through fire, that the earth is my support, that the water is my creator, and that the air is my nurse. I realize that our etheric streams are helped by the fire, by the feeling. This is the prelude to "thinking the will" and "willing the thinking".

6. In regard to the nine beams in therapy

I visualize a total division into (1-2-3-4-5-6-7-8-9) "beams". The 9 light beams relate to the stage where we enter the cosmic and unifying "I". This is the total energy coming down from the 9 hierarchies of angels, the totality of the higher level of inhabitants of the spiritual world. In this way, I am part of a greater healing force.

7. Regarding the phenomena of turning around

In the 5th Lesson, we start with recapitulation, and then for the first time the turning around is touched upon. The first turning around, before entering the threshold, is described. The next will be after the crossing of the threshold in lesson 6. The Guardian of the threshold exclaims that when we go back into the physical

---

[26] The importance of the touch of the tips of the fingers agains the forces of the blood in darkness is described by Judith von Halle as the initiation way of the Templers in her book «Die Templer, Band I», ISBN 978-3-03769-041-3.

world we must follow its laws, which are different from those of the spiritual world. When we go back, we must go with our thinking in the earth element, with the feeling in the water element, and with the will in the air element. At this point we may fear our old animal-like thinking but, for me, I feel sorrow.

To avoid this, we must moderate our will by thinking in the earth. Likewise, the feeling must be moderated by being awake in the water, and the thinking must be moderated by experiencing the will being awakened in the air. It is in this way that all becomes once again mingled: thinking to feeling, thinking to earth, will to air and thinking.

What is most interesting, however, is that when I come back into the physical and look back at the spiritual world, I have to push to get behind the thought of it. This is especially so when I still want to go back into the spiritual, as the Spirit-World always lies hidden behind my physical thoughts. This is when I need to have understanding and compassion for human pain (for the physical world), so that I do not fall into an illusion of false thinking.

Furthermore, I must again feel love for the physical world so that feeling does not also become illusionary. Finally, my will must feel the will of God in order for me not to be corrupted when coming back into the physical world.

In summary, I believe we need *Faith, Hope and Love* to purify our *Willing, Thinking and Feeling*.

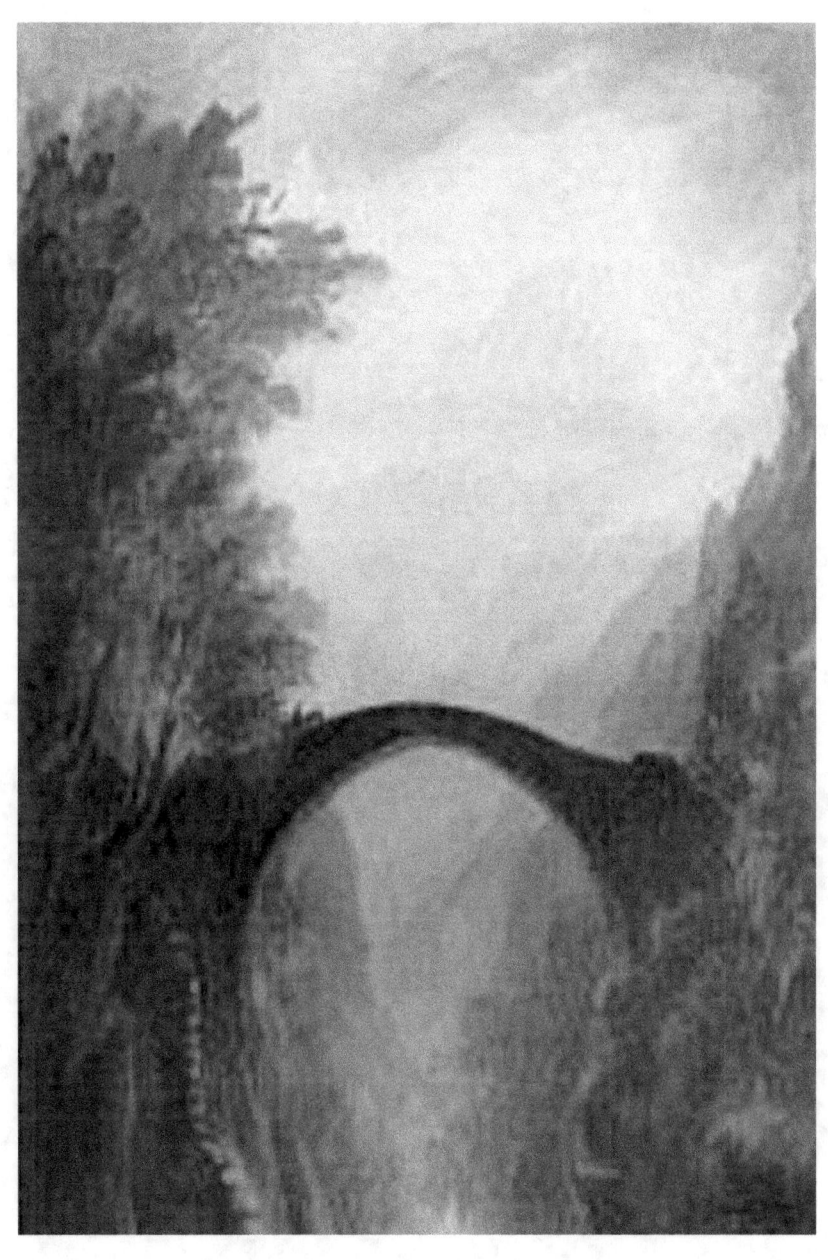

Chapter 4:

The Spiritual Pulse
The primary tool of Spiritual Medicine

Traditional Chinese Medicine and The Pulse

The aspect of pulse diagnosis as part of an acupuncture protocol is complex. Over thousands of years, it has undergone a metamorphosis as a result of a division of TCM into two often fundamentally opposed concepts. The first concept revolves around what is termed *eight-principle theory*. These principles are bipolar in nature and are guided by the decision as to what the physician should prescribe as an herbal formula. The patient is evaluated based on the following eight criteria:

1. Is the global picture of the patient Yin? (interior, cold, deficient)
2. Is the global picture of the patient Yang? (exterior, hot, excess)
3. Is the disease deeply imbedded and chronic (interior)?
4. Is the disease superficial and acute (exterior)?
5. Is the disease one of excess?
6. Is the disease one of deficiency?
7. Is the disease cold?
8. Is the disease hot?

The physician then uses the *four examinations* (listening, looking, touching, and smelling) to determine an appropriate herbal protocol to address the findings of these exams.

The exam that we shall focus on is that of touch, of which

taking the pulse plays a pivotal role. In addition to finding the answer to the above eight questions, the pulse can also help us determine the nature of what TCM calls the *4 fundamental substances* they see as critical to the functioning of the organism:

1. What is the nature of the fundamental substance of Yin (ie: estrogen)?
2. What is the nature of the fundamental substance of Yang (ie: thyroxin)?
3. What is the nature of the fundamental substance of Blood (ie: RBC s)?
4. What is the nature of the fundamental substance of Fluid? (joint fluid)?

In order to take the pulse, the physician places his fingers on the radial artery of the patient's left and right wrist. Depicted below is the position of where the pulse is taken. Note that the pulses on each wrist have a positional dependence, as each of the practitioner's second third and fourth finger can access the health of a specific meridian-organ of Chinese medicine.

In addition, the pulse will reveal several global aspects of the patient. In this case, the practitioner will check if the pulse is rapid (heat) or slow (cold), strong in force verses only slightly perceptible (excess vs deficiency), and more subjective qualities that denote specific organ involvement. This would include a wiry quality (as if you were feeling a guitar string) of a liver imbalance or the rolling action of a spleen imbalance likened to a wave under your finger. With this information, the diagnostician prepares a formula that would address these abnormal characteristics.

The other field of TCM that has evolved from a completely different construct is termed *five-element acupuncture*. This field of knowledge is based more on the aspects of selecting acupuncture points to balance the patient rather than the administration of herbal concoctions. Basically, the organ meridian processes are placed in categories analogous to the elements found in nature listed as Fire, Earth, Metal, Water and Wood. This form of acupuncture also requires feeling the pulse at the radial arteries of the wrists, but pays much more attention to the *relative* strength of each position of the pulse along the length of that artery. The practitioner concerns himself more with where the weakest pulse is found and how it compares to the other organ/meridians that are being accessed. This latter technique is the aspect of TCM that I learned when I studied acupuncture.

For veterinary alternative practitioners, attempting to take the pulse on the radial artery of our patients can be problematic. Fortunately, I discovered how to apply the technique of *surrogate* pulse diagnosis. adapting the techniques of kinesiology, which recognizes that the energy of the practitioner can merge with that of the patient, I found that if I took my own pulse at the relative positions described above and, at the same moment, made contact with the etheric energy of the patient, my pulse would temporarily take on the relative deficiencies and excesses of the animal being examined. However, in order to master this method, we must take on and develop the teachings that I shall present in this book.

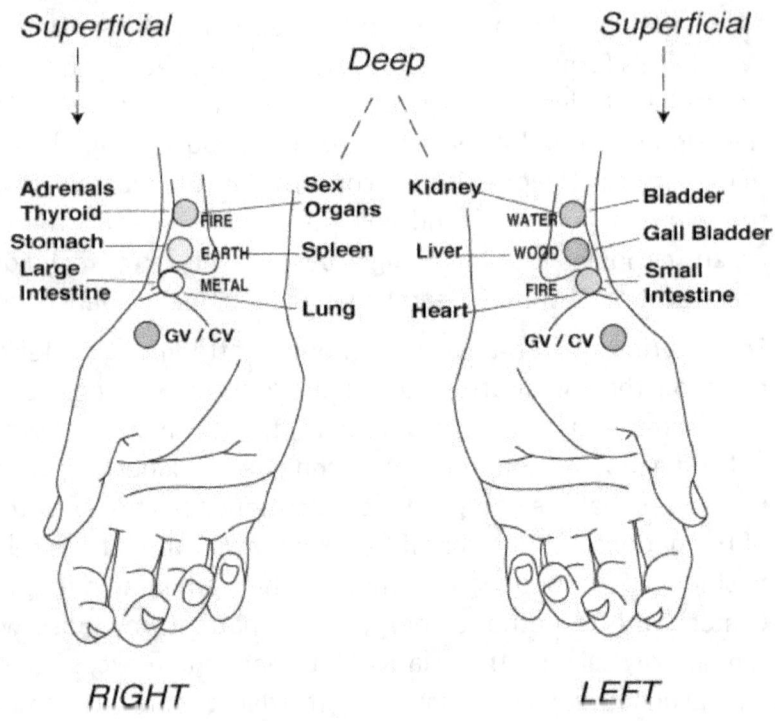

Positions of the organ/meridians on the radial arteries

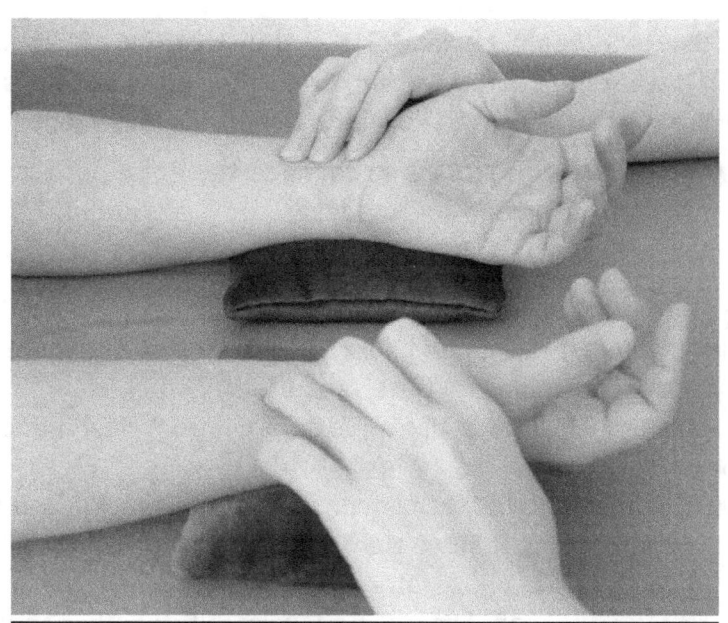

pulse diagnosis

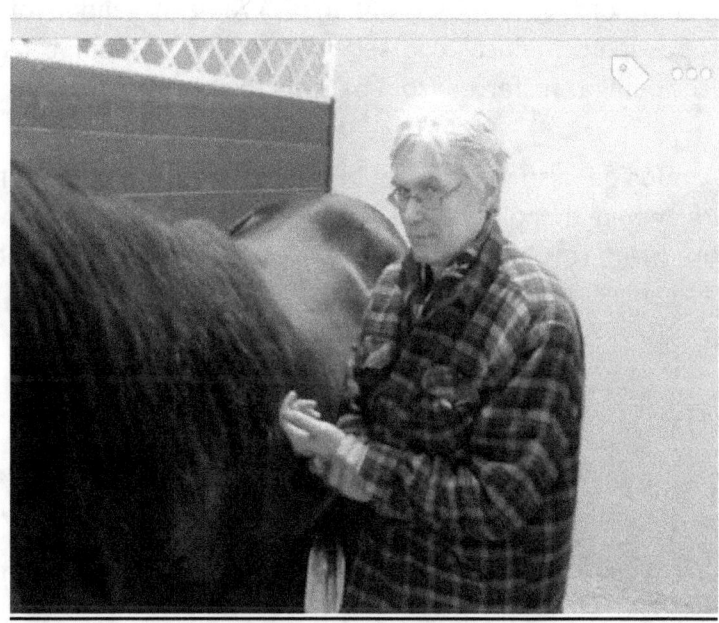

Surrogate Pulse diagnosis

In order to prepare better for the translocation of diseases, which is what the Chinese system prefer, the pulse positions are also changed, as well as the construction of the 5 elements.

How the Yellow emperors also changed the Pulse-positions to accomplish his deeds.

In hundreds of years before the Yellow Emperor changed the medical system, the Chinese had a 12-element system, where man and woman (Yang and Yin) were separated.
The pulse—diagnosis was also quite different from after the Yellow Emperor.
In creating the 5-elements the main change was that Yin and Yang was put together in the same element, and also both the heart and the pericardium was put together.
This resulted in man and woman was put together, and all differences between them were concealed.

This is, according to Dr. Johannes Weinzirl, leader of the anthroposophic medical courses in Chechia, a main cause of diseases being transferred from parents to children.

This confusion also happened in the 70-ties of the European culture, when the differences between man and woman were obscured, and resulted in massive waves of translocated diseases, such as cancer.

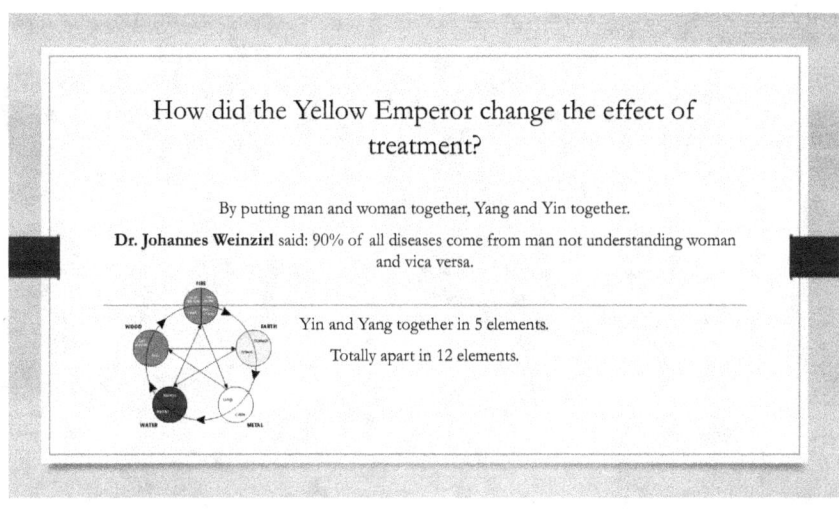

Also in pulse-diagnosis the same deceit was fulfilled. Before the time of the Yellow Emperor the positions of the Yin and the Yang, the female and the male, were far apart. Now they also were put together at the wrist of the human being, bringing man and woman together as if they were the same, as if they were one, thus preparing for the possibility of translocation.

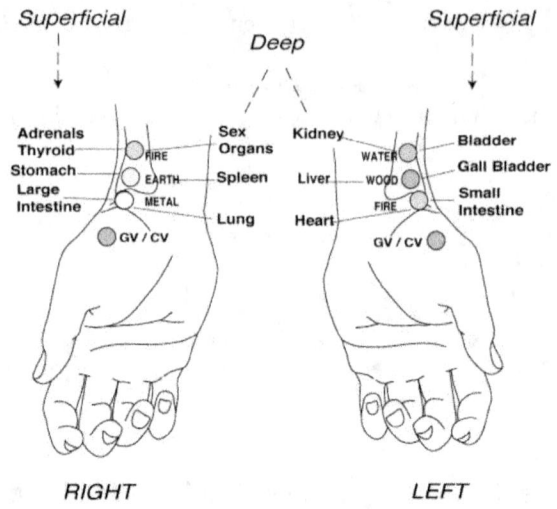

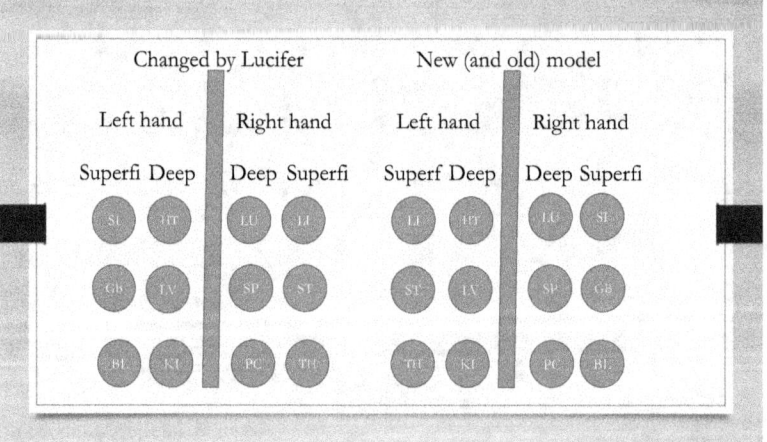

Here we see how the nowadays used system of pulse-diagnosis must be changed in the same way as the 5-elements has to be changed.

In the system that is usually used man and woman are placed together.

This must be changed, so that man is on the other hand of the woman.

In the "new model" we see that all the Yin/Yang pairs are broken up, and that each part of the pair is on the other hand, just as you will later see that we must do to the 5-elements.

The Pulse as an Exercise Toward Spiritual Development

For those readers versed in these traditional concepts of Chinese Pulse Diagnosis, the description I shall now present regarding pulse diagnosis will appear quite foreign. In my experience, taking the pulse is a precursor for an initiation into the spiritual world. What I am about to teach will be especially useful for those alternative practitioners who are acupuncturists, for this can be their way to access the experience necessary to evoke Christ consciousness.

When I started to teach pulse diagnosis to my students, I thought that it would be easy for them to monitor the pulse diagnostic patterns in their patients. I thought it was just a simple and straight forward method. Therefore, I was astonished when very few were able to master this technique. At the time, I had no explanation for this phenomenon.

I later discovered the reason. The pulse I was feeling was not obtained by my physical senses. The pulse I was looking for was etheric in nature and its true imbalance could only be found by my spiritual senses. My understanding that I always entered the spiritual world when taking a pulse did not come to my conscious attention until much later in life

Now that we have learned the path to initiation as described by Rudolf Steiner, we can be reminded of the similarities between his path and the method in which I proceed with my diagnostic exam. As I now realize that it is a doorway into the spiritual world, this method will also help us obtain the tools necessary to develop our spiritual organs.

The main skill we must learn, is the ability to become detached, as I have described previously as a state of not caring, not allowing the mind to wander, and not to act other than taking the pulse. In other words, pulse diagnosis must become as objective as possible with our total concentration directed toward the patient.

However, in the beginning, this state of indifference can be difficult to obtain. We are often distracted by a wandering or overly concerned mind. Therefore, we should strive to practice our pulse technique in an environment free of emotional obstacles such the judgement of observing colleagues in order to stay as relaxed as possible in both mind and body.

Because we are all anchored to the material world by an entanglement of our thinking, feeling and willing, our primary directive must always be in the forefront of our mind, to master the ability to separate these three soul qualities. Our mind may very well influence the result of our diagnostic work, just in the same way that the observer may influence an outcome as stated in quantum physics. Therefore, it is necessary that we maintain a neutral meditative state.[27]

As I have stated throughout this book, there is a close connection between the three directional vectors of the physical world and

---

[27] 'The secret life of Plants' authored by Tompkins and Bird: The authors discovered that plants respond favorably to the caregiver's positive attitude and negatively to negative emotions.

these three soul qualities. With this information, I formulated an effective technique to help with the separation.

To remind the reader, listed below, are the correlations between direction and each soul quality that I discussed earlier in this book:

1. Thinking = height, the upward direction (toward the cosmos).
2. Feeling = width, the outward direction (the expanses of our environment).
3. Will = depth, the downward direction (as if going into the earth).

Using this information, we can use our imagination and blur the delineation of the three dimensions of our physical world. In other words, we practice "fuzzy vision" by fading away, similar to a day dream where we become unaware of our surroundings as if in a state just before sleep.

I now realize that my spiritual inner life became richer because of my daily use of these techniques, and that developing the pulse can actually serve as a doorway to increased clairvoyance. The importance of this to the reader cannot be understated, as this exercise will provide a key to crossing the threshold.

Preparation for Taking the Pulse

Proper pulse taking requires a proper state of mind. This mind set can be described best as a state of day dreaming. When I began to learn the pulse, I struggled to create the conditions conducive to focused concentration and impartial objectivity. I created strict rituals. I had to be immaculately clean and free of physical needs, such as hunger and thirst. My environment required freedom from distractions. I created a situation optimal for a balanced state of mind. As with all learning, I slowly drifted from a state of conscious aptness to one of unconscious aptness, allowing me greater freedom to obtain a diagnosis without the preparations that I just described.

For the beginner, however, it is necessary to begin with the preparations that I described above. The first mind set one must adapt is a state of *"not caring"*. Of course, this first sounds as a kind of therapeutic blasphemy, implying an absence of empathy. Quite the contrary, it represents an emphatic thumb's up to faith. It is the opening of a door to the inward stream of information that the Christ impulse brings to us. Thus, the practitioner must not carry preconceptions of the causes of the disease, and shed all interest, anxiety or desire to reach a diagnosis or other prejudicial matter. This stance allows one to live in the exact moment of the pulse and nothing else.

Secondly, along with a sort of indifference, the practitioner must stay focused (*not mind wandering*). One should concentrate totally and exclusively on the patient. The rest of the world has to be blocked out during this procedure.

Finally, the practitioner should *"not act"*. This is actually the description of the achieved meditative state, when one seems to fade away, as if he were under the influence of a hypnotic suggestion. These are the qualities that create the alpha wave activity in the brain to increase. In anthroposophic terms, this is referred to as separating the soul faculties of thinking, feeling and willing[28].

In my experience, the soul faculty of feeling is the simplest to separate. Therefore, one can start the process by separating width from height and depth. This is done by using the tools of anthroposophic meditative techniques to induce a state of

---

[28] Academically, this change between the non-separation and the separation of the soul abilities is called a "noetic slippage". This slippage is a spiritual state where the mind changes between chaos and order, between light and darkness, between dioysian and apollonian, between the noetic and the chthonic.

daydreaming where one merges into the wide expanses of the surroundings. Imagine yourself listening to a boring lecture. This is the feeling of fading away. When thinking and willing are separated from feeling you feel as if you are floating, and you have no strength nor desire to will or think of anything. Often the sense of hearing will be muted by an internal ringing, and the color of the landscape will darken, taking on a violet hue. Many find themselves subconsciously tilting their head slightly to the right[29]

It is now at this point that we direct this separated and pure faculty of feeling to concentrate on the blood flowing in our fingertips from the heart and create a deep connection with our patient and his pulse. It is at this point that we are essentially inside that patient.

While we are learning these techniques, we must also keep in mind the difference between the laws of the physical world and those of the spiritual world. In the spiritual world, we are not bound by dimension and time. With that said, we can travel vast distances in the blink of an eye. We can move through time, as it is no longer absolute. Now a thought becomes an intention and an intention becomes a thing. This is the law of destiny as a reflection of our past and present karma.

---

[29] The **Elf-School** is open all year around in Reykjavik. It has been in operation for 28 years. Their unique curriculum revolves around understanding elemental beings including the hidden people, elves, Gnomes, dwarfs, fairies, trolls, mountain Spirits as well as other nature Spirits and mythical beings in Iceland and in other countries. The students in The Elf school also learn about the hundreds of Icelanders that have had personal contact with the elves. Many of them have been invited into the homes of the elves and the hidden people of Iceland and have often eaten food there and sometimes have even slept there one or more nights. The argument that the elves and hidden people of Iceland have saved hundreds of lives of Icelanders through the centuries is explored and explained to the students, as well as how this strange friendship between our world and the many other worlds or dimensions can and does exist.

As long as we are in the grip of the entanglement of these soul faculties, we cannot detect the energetic changes necessary to truly heal our patients. There are no shortcuts. Despite the descriptive attempts of the use of psychotropic agents by many to induce this state, these methods create a false presentment of the spiritual world.

The hands as spiritual organs:

Another correlation between Spiritual Science and my development of pulse diagnosis was evident in the lecture given by Rudolf Steiner on August 26, 1912 in Munich. This is what he said regarding the hands as spiritual sense organs:

> "The etheric organs of the hands are true spiritual organs. The etheric organs expressed in the hands and their functions, work far more intuitively, more spiritually, and perform a far higher task than is accomplished by the etheric brain. Whoever has made progress in these matters will say that the brain with its etheric basis is in effect by far the least skillful of the spiritual organs man bears within him.
>
> The spiritual activities connected with the organs underlying the hands, but incompletely expressed in the hands and their functions, serve a far higher, more spiritual kind of knowledge and observation. These organs can lead into the super-sensible world and can occupy themselves with our perception and orientation there. A spiritual seer may express this, somewhat surprisingly but accurately, by saying that the human brain is a most clumsy organ for research in the spiritual world, and that the hands, or the spiritual basis of the

hands, are far more interesting and significant organs for gaining knowledge of the world and are certainly far more skillful organs than the brain. Not much is gained on the way to initiation by advancing from the use of the physical brain to a free use of the etheric brain. The difference is not great between what may be achieved through purified, intuitive brain thinking, and regulated spiritual working in the etheric spiritual counterpart of the brain. The difference is much greater between what our hands accomplish in the world, and what can be done by the etheric part that is the spiritual basis of the hands, than the physical brain. On the path of initiation not much development of the etheric brain is necessary since it is not a particularly important organ. But the etheric basis of the hands is connected with the activity of the lotus flower in the region of the heart, as you will learn in my book; "Knowledge of the Higher Worlds and Its Attainment".

This lotus flower pours out its rays of force in such a way as to build up the organism that, at the stage at which physical man now stands, exists in an incomplete form in the hands and their functions. Though it may sound strange, yet it is true that the least skillful organ for spiritual investigation is the brain, since it is the least capable of development. On the other hand, entirely new perspectives are opened out when we consider other apparently subordinate organs."

From the Head to the Throat to the heart

As the years passed and my skills intensified, I started to develop my spiritual sense organs. The first spiritual organ was the one of sight. I began to see the etheric energy of myself, my patients, and all living things. I could see it connecting between the trees, then among the animals and among the people.

In the beginning, I felt that my observations originated from the sensory center in the back of the brain, I saw that this energy flowed in a downward direction, traversing my arm, and entering my fingers to act as a source for both diagnosis and healing as I applied the needles to my patients. But then it started to wander. First it wandered towards the heart, then the spine, and then slowly spread throughout the entire body. The observations also became enlarged from an intellectual observation, to an immediate knowledge of past, present and future from observing what I was feeling from the pulse. The direction of this observation, which now had become knowledge, also changed. In the beginning, the direction of the information streamed from the surroundings or the patient towards me, but then it started to go both ways, as if the patient also received treatment at the same time as I was diagnosing. The observation also enlarged in space, as it came to include also the astral part of the patient's make up. This part was seen as a light flowing area, mingled together with the darker etheric energy. Then the observation started to move in time, to where past, present and future became one.

The first picture shown below, demonstrates what I spiritually see in the head of a beginner taking the pulse. The soul qualities of thinking, feeling and willing are entangled. In this way, the thought processes are consumed with daily living, leaving little etheric energy for pulse diagnosis or treating the patient

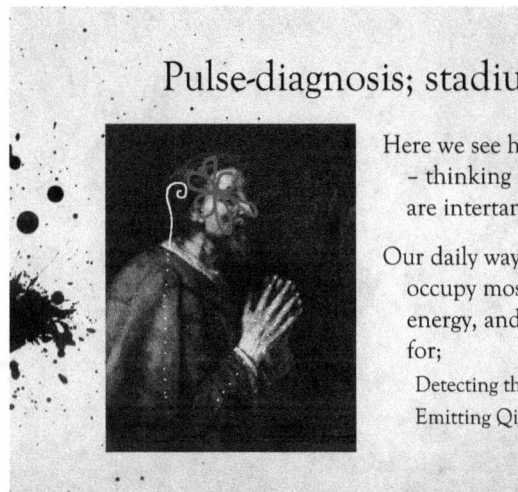

Pulse-diagnosis; stadium I

Here we see how willing – thinking and feeling are intertangled

Our daily way of thinking occupy most of the energy, and leave little for;
- Detecting the pulse
- Emitting Qi

However, as discussed in the previous chapter, with training, years of practice, and correct meditation, the soul faculties begin to separate, allowing the stream of energy from the head to strengthen. This ultimately improves the ability of the practitioner to both diagnose and treat.

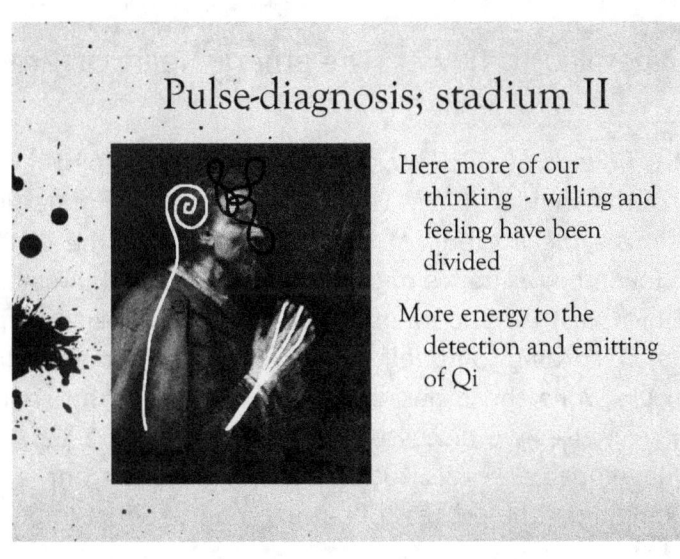

Pulse-diagnosis; stadium II

Here more of our thinking - willing and feeling have been divided

More energy to the detection and emitting of Qi

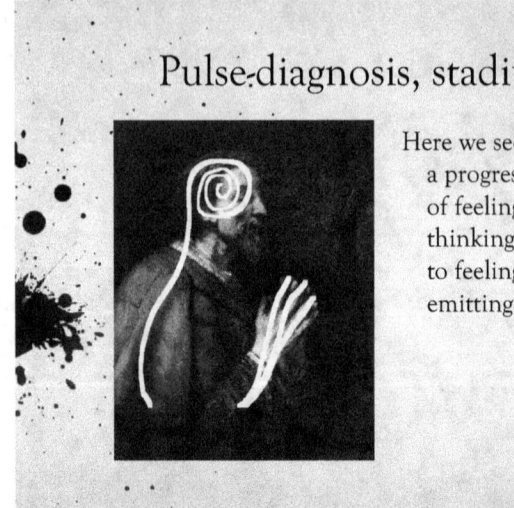

Pulse-diagnosis, stadium III

Here we see the effect of a progressed dividing of feeling – willing and thinking; much energy to feeling the pulse and emitting Qi

As thinking, feeling and willing become disengaged from one another, the etheric energy that is centered in the head begins to move downward. This movement is closely linked to the development of Christianity when Christ appeared on earth. This is the movement toward the heart.

The 12 petal lotus flower: The etheric Heart Organ

The lotus flowers of anthroposophy represent the spiritual sense organs of the soul faculties. The twelve-petal lotus, in particular, characterizes the makeup of the heart chakra as the center of selfless love, the residence of the Christ impulse and the eventual source of a vast etheric energy that we can utilize to help our patients. According to Rudolf Steiner, six of these petals already exist in us, while the other six are formed using the six moral esoteric exercises we discussed in chapter 4. The 12-petal lotus when developed, reveals to the budding clairvoyant a deep understanding of the process of nature and the Christ impulse.

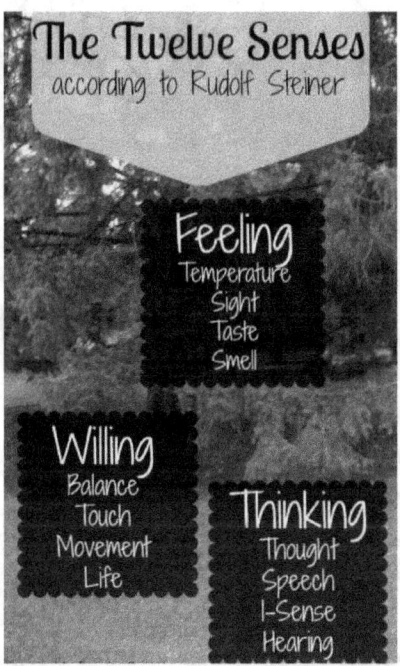

Rudolf Steiner says the following about this development.

> "When esoteric development has progressed so far that the lotus flowers begin to stir, much has already been achieved by the student which can result in the formation of certain quite definite currents and movements in his etheric body. The object of this development is the formation of a kind of center in the region of the physical heart, from which radiate currents and movements in the greatest possible variety of colors and forms. The center is in reality not a mere point, but a most complicated structure, a most wonderful organ. It glows and shimmers with every shade of color and displays forms of great symmetry, capable of rapid transformation. Other forms and streams of color radiate from this organ to the other parts of the body, and

beyond it to the astral body, completely penetrating and illuminating it. The most important of these currents flow to the lotus flowers. They permeate each petal and regulate its revolutions; then streaming out at the points of the petals, they lose themselves in outer space. The higher the development of a person, the greater the circumference to which these rays extend.

The twelve-petal lotus flower has a particularly close connection with this central organ. The currents flow directly into it and through it, proceeding on the one side to the sixteen and the two-petal lotus flowers, and on the other, the lower side, to the flowers of eight, six and four petals. It is for this reason that the very greatest care must be devoted to the development of the twelve-petal lotus, for an imperfection in the latter would result in irregular formation of the whole structure. The above will give an idea of the delicate and intimate nature of esoteric training, and of the accuracy needed if the development is to be regular and correct. It will also be evident beyond doubt that directions for the development of super sensible faculties can only be the concern of those who have themselves experienced everything which they propose to awaken in others, and who are unquestionably in a position to know whether the directions they give lead to the exact results desired. If the student follows the directions that have been given him, he introduces into his etheric body currents and movements which are in harmony with the laws and the evolution of the world to which he belongs. Consequently, these instructions are reflections of the great laws of cosmic evolution. They consist of the above-mentioned and similar exercises in meditation and concentration, which, if correctly practiced, produce the results described. The student must at certain times let these instructions permeate his soul with their content, so that he is inwardly entirely filled with it. A simple start is *made with a view to the deepening of the logical activity of the mind and the producing of an inward intensification of thought. Thought is thereby made free and independent of all sense impressions and experiences; it is concentrated in one point, which is held entirely under control. Thus, a preliminary center is formed for the currents of the etheric body. This center is not yet in the region of the heart but in the head, and it appears to the clairvoyant as the point of departure for movements and currents. No esoteric training can be successful which does not first create this center. If the latter were first formed in the region of the heart the aspiring clairvoyant would doubtless obtain glimpses of the higher worlds but would lack all true insight into the connection between these higher worlds and the world of our senses. This, however, is an unconditional necessity for man at the present stage of evolution. The clairvoyant must not become a visionary; he must retain a firm footing upon the earth.*

The center in the head, once duly fixed, is then moved lower down, to the region of the larynx. This is effected by further exercises in concentration. Then the currents of the etheric body radiate from this point and illuminate the astral space surrounding the individual.

Continued practice enables the student to determine for himself the position of this etheric body. Hitherto this position depends upon external forces proceeding from the physical body. Through further development the student is able to turn his etheric body to all sides. This faculty is affected by currents moving approximately along both hands and centred in the two-petal lotus in the region of the eyes. All this is made possible through the radiations from the larynx assuming round forms, of which a number flow to the two-petal lotus and thence form undulating currents along the hands. As a further development, these currents branch out and ramify in the most delicate manner and become, as it were, a kind of web which then encompasses the entire etheric body as though with a network. Whereas hitherto the etheric body was not closed to the outer world, so that the life currents from the universal ocean of life flowed freely in and out, these currents now have to pass through this membrane. Thus, the individual becomes sensitive to these external streams; they become perceptible to him.

And now the time has come to give the complete system of currents and movements its center situated in the region of the heart. This again is effected by persevering with the exercises in concentration and meditation; and at this point also the stage is reached when the student becomes gifted with the inner word. All things now acquire a new significance for him. They become as it were, spiritually audible in their innermost self, and speak to him of their essential being. The currents described above place him in touch with the inner being of the world to which he belongs. He begins to mingle his life with the life of his environment and can let it reverberate in the movements of his lotus flowers."

Concentration on the heart

Before I take the pulse, I begin by my spiritual preparation. This consist of a mixture of:

- the northern stream
- and the southern stream.

First, to get into the spiritual world, I chose the northern technique.

I "vanish" into the surrounding nature, just as described in Parsifal or in The Kalavala. This vanishing causes the tight bond between the etheric body and the astral body to loosen somewhat. Then I enter the spiritual world.

Being there I chose what soul-faculty or body-art I want to work with. I then chose the heart, and from the heart I separate the feeling from the thinking and the willing, and with this decision I enter the southern stream or technique.

As I am separating and isolating the soul faculty of "feeling", I discard my own ego-centered feelings, and replace them with a sort of cosmic analogue. A global love for everything. Later, when I consider the diagnosis (thinking) and treatment (willing), I also leave the other two faculties, either feeling and willing or thinking and feeling, and try to use only one of the divine forces.

However, when I first enter the diagnostic process, I enter my feeling force through my own heart, and concentrate on the heart of the patient. I visualize that I am creating a tunnel or portal between my own heart and that of the patient. I enter this tunnel only with my feeling, leaving both the thinking and the willing outside. In going towards the heart of the patient, I now imagine the 12-layer microsystem of sheaths that begins at the physical skin of the patient and ends in the inside of his spiritual heart.

I first picture going through the 8 layers of the body of the patient, and then into the 4 layers of the heart, a total of 12 layers. The 8th layer is where we move past the body to enter the 9th layer, represented by the endocardium, and enter the realm of the heart, the spiritual center of man. To go from the material realm of the body and into the spiritual realm of the heart.

Most students stop before the 8th layer and are unable to enter the heart. It appears that this step requires the presence of a strong and determined will in order to push past this level. It is easiest to understand how to accomplish this if we first learn to visualize these 12 layers of the body as listed below

1. The outer layers (1-2) relate to the astral body.
2. The next (3rd-4th) to the material body (3rd being our own physical, material body, 4th parasitic material bodies).
3. The 5th-6th-7th-8th relate to the etheric (the 4 ethers) body (the 7th touching the pericardium and the 8th touching the endocardium), where we leave the material world ……
4. The inner layers (9th-10th-11th-12th) are within the heart, and relate to the "I"; the lower I (9th), the middle I (10th), the higher I (11th) and the cosmic I (the Christ consciousness) (12th), where we are in the middle of the heart, the lamb (ram), the Christ consciousness.

The 12 layers of the pulse

Between the skin (actually outside the skin) there are 12 layers, or depths, of which disease may be diagnosed (or treated)

- The outer layer (1-2) relate to the astral body
- The next (3-4) to the material body (3 being our own material body, 4. parasitic material bodies)
- The 5-6-7-8 to the etheric (the 4 ethers) body (the 7. touching the pericardium and the 8. touching the endocardium), where we leave the material world ……
- The inner (9-10-11-12) are within the heart, and relate to the "I"; the lower I (9), the middle I (10), the higer I (11) and the cosmic I (the Christ conciousness) (12), where we are in the middle of the heart, the lamb (ram), the Christ conciousness.

When we are in the middle of the heart, we should imagine standing at a cross. This cross is a little different in a man, horse and dog.

In this picture below, I have tried to illustrate these crosses.

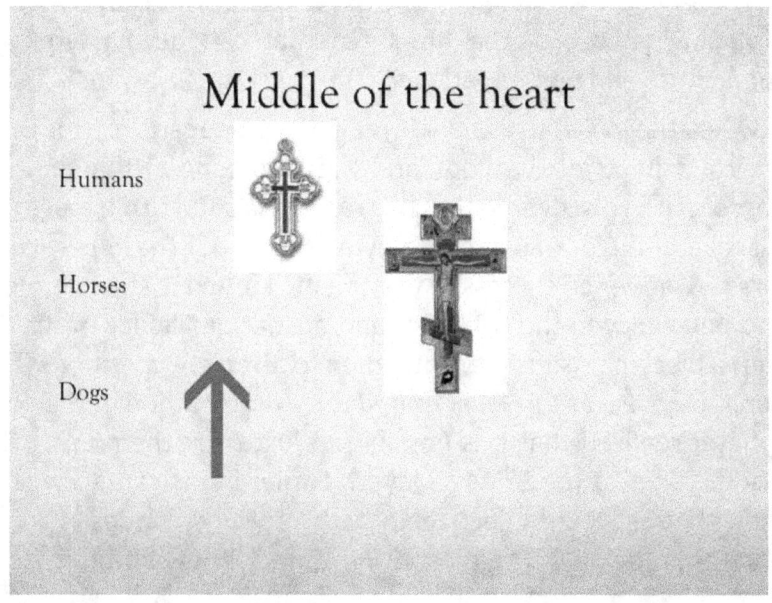

On the way through the 12 layers we may diagnose, experience and/or treat the different aspects present in these layers concerning diseases or spiritual realities. For example, the two outer layers relate to the astral body of the patient. These layers reflect feelings and emotions. If we stop at this layer, and take the pulse here, we get an emotional diagnosis.

The 3rd and 4th layers both reflect the physical body. The third layer being our own physical body and the fourth related to the material bodies of parasites that exist within us. If we stop evaluating the pulse at the 3ʳᵈ or 4ᵗʰ layer we will be able to diagnose the imbalances present in the physical body. Exploring the pulse at the 4ᵗʰ layer is especially interesting as here we can detect the presence of both physical and energetic parasites in the body of the patient.

The layers where most beginners seem to stop is at the etheric level, located between the 5ᵗʰ and the 8ᵗʰ layer. This is the location of healing energy of the life force that can be activated by acupuncture and homeopathy.

Between the 8ᵗʰ and the 9ᵗʰ layer lies the departure from the physical aspects of the body and the beginning of the spiritual heart organ. I discovered that this region is useful to diagnose the presence of a blockage created by a toxic scar. These particular scars can prevent a successful treatment. I found that when there is no deficiency in the 8ᵗʰ layer, and a clear deficiency in the 9ᵗʰ layer, a blocking scar is present. I then focused my intention while taking the pulse at this level to *find* the exact location of the scar, but later realized that it is possible to just *treat* them using the pulse findings at the 9ᵗʰ ⁻ 12ᵗʰ layer. Earlier in my career, when I found them I would inject them with procaine, as described in neural therapy by Dr. Ferdinand Hünecke.[30] I now find this to be

---

[30] The father of neural therapy: The idea underlying the therapy is that "interference fields" (*Störfelder*) at certain sites of the body are responsible for a type of electric energy that causes illness. The fields can be disrupted by injection, allowing the body to heal. The practice originated in 1925 when Ferdinand Huneke, a German surgeon, used a newly launched pain drug that contained procaine (a local anaesthetic) on his sister who had severe intractable migraines. Instead of using it intramuscularly as recommended he injected it intravenously and the migraine attack stopped immediately. He and his brother Walter subsequently used Novocaine in a similar way to treat a variety of ailments. In 1940 Ferdinand Huneke injected the painful shoulder of a woman who also had an osteomyelitis in her leg, which at that time (before antibiotics) threatened her with amputation. The shoulder pain improved somewhat but the leg wound became itchy. On injecting the leg wound the shoulder pain vanished

unnecessary, as I have learned to always treat using the findings when focused on the 12th layer.

I feel that the four layers within the heart itself are of immense importance. From here we may diagnose and treat diseases from the spiritual realm of the patient. This, in my opinion is the best hope to be able to cure the patient

The inner (9th - 10th - 11th - 12th) are within the heart, and relate to the I; the lower I (9th), the middle I (10th), the higher I (11th) and the cosmic I (the Christ consciousness) (12th), where we are in the middle of the heart, where the lamb (ram), the Christ consciousness resides. When we treat from the middle of the heart, we are in the deepest spiritual realm, and here the usual stumbling blocks are gone.

After going through the 12 layers of the patient, I have to choose the appropriate microsystem to use in my treatment; the system of 2 (yin and yang), 3 (thinking, feeling, willing), 4 (which sheath), 5 (which element), 7 (which chakra or 12 (which meridian).

The Mystery of the Turning Around

Just before the diagnosis is done, I come to the mystery of "The turning around", re-entering the physical realm for the first time, and returning from the spiritual. Re-entering the physical is necessary to see if the decisions I have made concerning the therapy are correct. Here, I often feel sadness for the patient, in seeing his karma and the effect of his disease. At this point, I mingle all ways of therapy in my imagination, to decide which one is the best. However, I look for the area of health, or the "Christ"

---

immediately – a reaction he called the "phenomenon of seconds" (*Sekundenphänomen*).

within the body, focusing on one of the anatomical middle points.

The Second Turning Around

After finding this point, I must let the will of God come forth. I accomplish this by treating or stimulating the middle alone or in addition with a more specific therapy. This is the point that I perform the second turning around.

When I found Steiner's description of the development of an initiate in "Umrisse der Okkulten Wissenschaft" translated as "An outline of Occult Science", I found this to be an accurate description of what I had experienced during the last 29 years.

As Steiner predicted, this moment finally came for me. The center of my focus moved from the head to the heart. But with this development, my "old" methods of treatment stopped working. I came to realize that I had to develop a new method that could match my spiritual growth. I discovered that I had to alter the focus of my treatment from the deficiency point determined by pulse diagnosis, to the middle point found by the use of my spiritual senses. Furthermore, I recognized the need to treat my patient as part of a co-joined group rather than as an individual. As the Bible states, "Where there is a gathering of two or more in the name of the Lord".

Going Back Through Time Using the Pulse

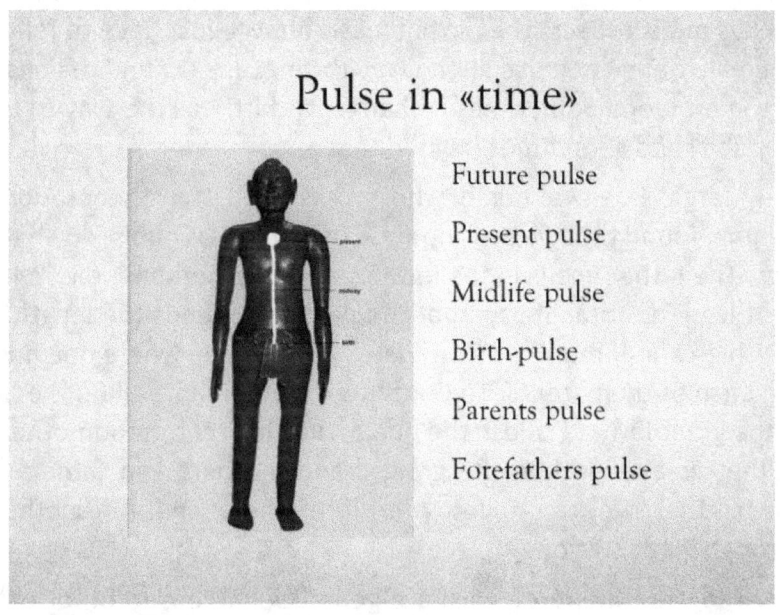

As time operates differently in the spirit world, we can use our ability to take the spiritual pulse to evaluate the patient at any point of time in their life cycle. We accomplish this by taking the pulse and as we enter into the spiritual world, we concentrate on our own heart and then enter into the heart of the patient. We visualize going all the way to the 12th layer where we are at the deepest present pulse. There we then find the most deficient pulse. Holding this deficient pulse, we scan the midsection of the patient beginning at the top of the sternum, and let our eyes travel distally along the midline. If the deficient pulse disappears, let us say midway to the Os pubis, the cause the disease, started midway in life.

The total pulse-picture will change radically when in our mind we travel along the midline distally, which is going back in time. The distance between the center of the heart and Os pubis resembles the total life span. Midway resembles midway in life. The Os pubis reflects the birth, and so on. We just have to follow the main deficient pulse all the way through life, to find the onset of the problem. Sometimes it changes at birth, all the way to the Os pubis, and sometimes beyond that.

Margit Buen, a nurse who works with trans-generational trauma, found that we can continue below the Os pubis, down the legs. The father line is in the left leg, and the mother line is in the right leg. The total life span of the parents extends the length of the thigh and femur, and terminates at the knee, where one finds the birth of the parents. To Continue, in the tibia, we find the life of the grandfathers, and in the fibula, the life of the grandmothers. In the tarsals, we find the great-grand mothers and fathers. It seems that we can follow the forefathers and foremothers through 7 generations.

The treatment of this pre-generational onset of disease through different forms of trauma (like war, prison, concentration camps, rape, murder and so on) is to put a needle, with intention and knowledge, exactly at the point of the onset of the disease, at the starting point of the deficiency.

A little deeper understanding of the four "ethers", explained through studying a Norwegian Stave-church.

First some descriptions of the structure of the "Stave-church".

The first thing I observed as I approached the stave-church, well after activating "my" etheric sense of clarity, was that the entire stake church consisted of four circles or "layers," much like in a puff pastry, of elemental beings. These moved in opposite directions, and there was no communication between them. The lower layer, which moved with the sun, was the elemental beings belonging to the earth element, Gnomes, they express the life-etheric-element.
The next layer consisted of Undine-like elemental beings belonging to the water element, expressing the Chemical Ether.
The next layer consisted of Sylphide-like elemental beings belonging to the air element, expressing the Light-ether.
The next, last and uppermost layer consisted of Salamander-like elementary beings belonging to the fire (heat) element, and is the expression of the warmth-etheric-ether.
I saw this in the spire and in the small sphere that was placed on top of the spire.
Most anthroposophists know what we call the etheric body, the transcendental force structure that nourishes and allows us to grow, but even when growth is over, our thoughts and our memory carry.

These etheric forces consist of four parts:

- Life-ether, the earth element, forms the structure of the physical world.
- Chemical ether, the water element, forms the basis for "metabolism".
- Light-ether, the air element, forms the basis for feelings.

• Heat eaters, which form the basis of our ego and belong to the element of fire.

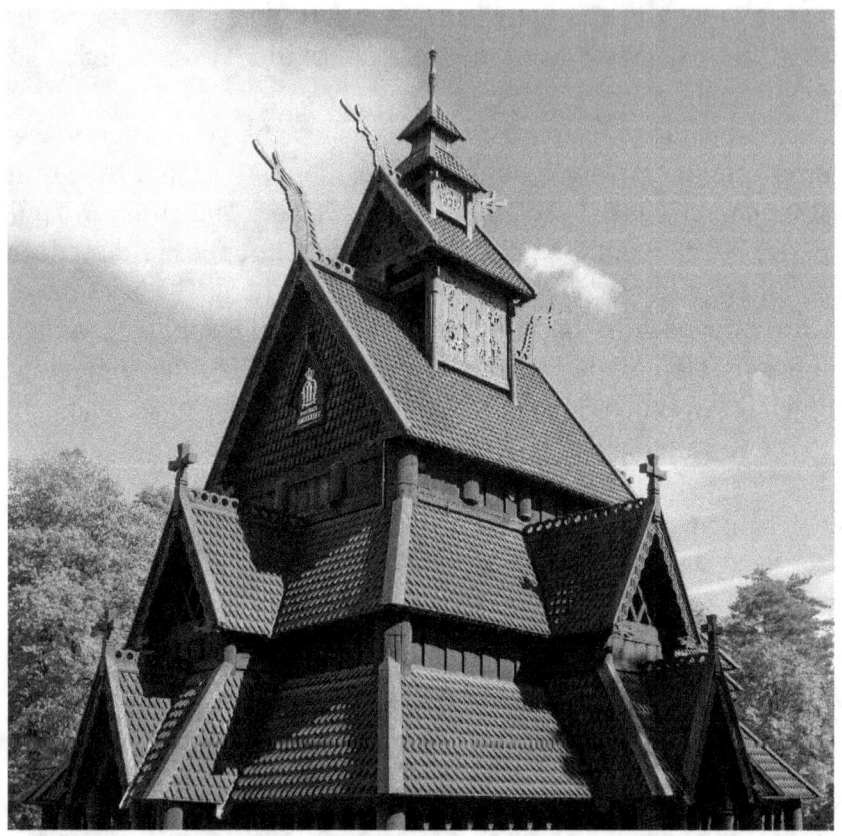

As we entered the stake church, we can see the symbols of the four ethers drawn into the inner walls of the stave-church, in four layers.

Squares expressing the Gnomes, or the Life-center.
Crescents expressing the Undines, or the Chemical Ether.
Triangles expressing the Sylphides, or Light-ether.
Circles or spheres expressing the Salamanders or the warmth-ether.

These symbols were drawn in circles around the inside walls of the stake church, just as I saw the elementary beings move outside the church.

The Effect of the Therapist on the outcome of treatment

I have repeatedly experienced the disappointment in many of my students when they admit that the methods that I taught often failed to work for them. Of course, this was rather confusing for me until I had the epiphany that the positive effects of my therapeutic methods were directly dependent on the level of spiritual development of the therapist enlisting such techniques.

To exemplify this point, I would like to share an experience I had with two of my French colleagues, Jaques Beneviste and Luc Montagniers. The former, became famous for a large volume of work he did on an attempt to prove the scientific validity of homeopathy. Sadly, he and his work was discredited by a group of doctors known as the "quackbusters". Following his exact protocols, they were unable to get the same results.

I came up with two possible explanations with reference to the tenants of this book. First, without being in the objective meditative state to enter the spiritual world, we can negatively impact the results of our attempts by our entanglement of feeling, thinking and willing. Beneviste, being a practitioner with the ability to individualize these soul qualities, was able to manifest the positive outcome that homeopathy can provide.

The second possibility of Beneviste's failure may relate to the second book of this trilogy. The effect of demons. From my own spiritual investigation, I have personally visualized that each homeopathic remedy has an accompanying elemental being, the spirit of the material substance.

A summary of how to use Thinking, Feeling and Willing in the medical treatment of patients.

Thinking must be used in the initial stage of the diagnosis of any patient, both animal and man. We must inquire about the nature of the disease, make our observations and determine how to perform the treatment. Is surgery needed, is the horse dangerous, can the dog bite us, do we need any medications and so on?

Then we proceed to the method of separating Thinking, Feeling and Willing as described in this book. When we have reached this state of mind, we proceed to focus on the soul faculty of Feeling, visualizing the heart, and diagnose the patient. Here is when we leave the thinking and willing behind. We imagine spiritually entering the 12th layer of our heart. We then imagine a tunnel from our heart to the heart of the patient. This tunnel traverses all 12 layers of the body to end at the center of the patient's heart.

Keeping are focus here, we make our diagnosis. Personally, I use the pulse-diagnosis to go through all the different processes of the body, both in the present time and in the past, however any modality of Spiritual diagnosis may be used whether it be homeopathy, kinesiology or any method that may give me the information I need. We can also go into the processes of the forefathers and foremothers, investigating the different physical, mental or spiritual traumas, and in doing this, we mentally organize the information that we have gathered. This is when we combine the Thinking with the Feeling.

When we have decided with our Thinking how to treat this disease, we again leave both the thinking and the feeling behind, and go into the Will power of the universe, which is to be found in the earth itself. This Will force must be used in the therapeutic part of the procedure. The focus of the therapist will then be in his limbs, his feet, or even in the earth beneath his feet. From this area, the force of Will is awakened, and this force will then stream up through the body. The path this force takes is not along the spine, as described in old traditions as the "Kundalini" force. This up-going stream should be found in front of the spine. The force in the spine is of the old world, related to Lucifer. The force of the new world is in the middle of the front of the body, related to Christ.

It is possible to experience this up-going stream as a dance between two snakes, one white and one black. This force must then enter the heart and mingle with the feeling, compassion and love for the patient, and, in fact, for the whole of humanity (if we activate the Kundalini force, this goes straight to the crown chakra, and does not stop at the level of the heart). This mingling often results in a feeling of Cosmic divine love, inhabiting the center of the heart. From this center, the healing force, now totally cleaned from any egoistic wish or intent, streams over into the patient through our hands and fingers. Here, directed by intentional thought that streams down from the head, the healing force works in the body by diminishing the power of the Demons. If this force is directed against the ahrimanic demon, the healing of the organic structures will begin. If it is directed against the luciferic demon, the pain and unpleasantness will diminish. If it is directed to the Middle, the Christ-Point or the Christ-filled gap between the two demons, both demons will pull back and start to dissolve or transform.

Spiritual Medicine

Part Two

Demons
The Faculty of Feeling

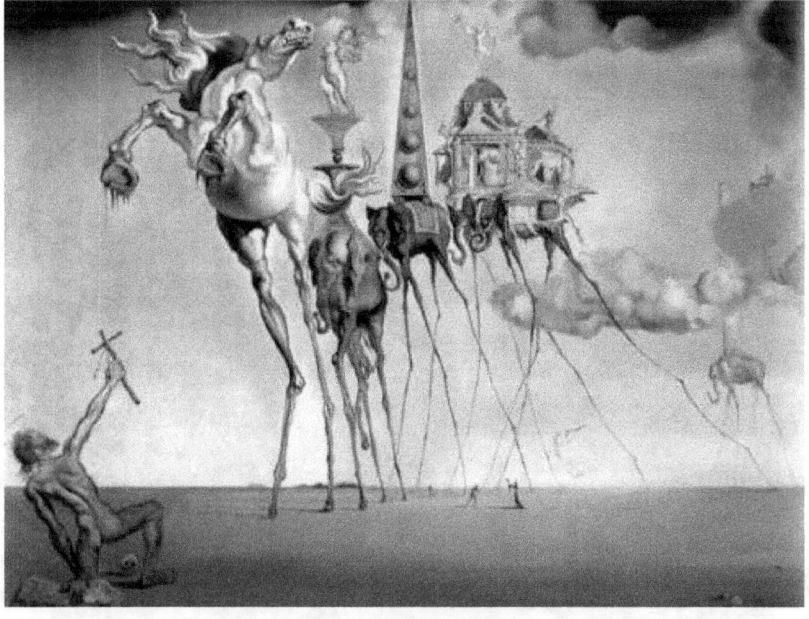

The holy St. Antonius temptation by Salvador Dali.[31]

---

[31] Representation of the demonic creatures of the 8th sphere or "planet of death." According to Steiner, it is where corrupt souls are dismantled to become elemental entities and share a world with insect like demons as shown above.

Chapter 5:

Demons, An Overview of Their Role in Spiritual Medicine

It began at a seminar in Worpswede, Germany. I was treating a horse using his Middle-Point and attempting to initiate the Christ-Consciousness in myself during the treatment. I then saw, with my spiritual eye, "something" emerging from the horse. This "something" swirled around inside the circle of observers. It behaved as if it was being trapped by these students. Then, suddenly, it disappeared into thin air. The most interesting part of this story was related to a sudden illness that one of the participants felt immediately after I released this "something" from the horse. Apparently, this student happened to attract a part of the "something" that was released. She went home after the seminar and, thanks to her therapist who quickly released what I now know to be a "partial pathological structure", was restored. I later realized that an entity had inserted itself in etheric level of her heart.

As will be shown throughout this book, this "something" lives and behaves as an individual and conscious entity. In other words, it is a demon. I know this term instils disbelief in many readers. I could have described these entities as pathological structures, but this would have been disingenuous. Therefore, I prefer to be honest and call it what I believe it to be.

Within the framework of an acupuncture construct, a tool I use the most in my practice, I further differentiated these demons as having a yin or yang quality[32]. In my perspective, I see ahrimanic type demons as representing the disorders that are Yin in nature and luciferic demons as demonstrating those of Yang. I have also discovered that these pathological demons emerge from the world of benign elemental beings. This virulent transformation is fueled by the misdeeds of our patients, and manifest as pathology when they gain entry into such susceptible beings.

What are Spirits?

As was discussed in the preface, it is of paramount importance that a healer not only considers treating humans and/or animals as separate beings, but rather as a part of a greater picture that includes the entire cosmos that is, by nature, spiritual. This spiritual world contains both good and evil, and in this particular book of my Trilogy, the emphasis will be in understanding the role of evil, which includes the presence of demons. I will also, in part three, *"Where 2 or 3 are Gathered",* contrast these sinister forces against the healing processes of good, represented by Christ.

However, these demons are only part of a greater "Spiritual World" also inhabited by benevolent spirits that do not influence a human's free will. The types of entities found in the higher world are varied. These spirits often exert a positive influence on man,

---

[32] Yin and yang: In Chinese philosophy, **this** describes the construct of how seemingly opposite or contrary forces may actually be complementary, interconnected, and interdependent in the natural world, and how they may give rise to each other as they interrelate. Many tangible dualities (such as light and dark, fire and water, expanding and contracting) are thought of as physical manifestations of the duality symbolized by yin and yang.

and include nature spirits, spirits of people who have died, and higher-level spirits such as angels.

Demons, on the other hand, have their own consciousness and effect humans in a malevolent way. They are created when the otherwise beneficial forces from Ahriman and Lucifer are distorted from the thoughts and misdeeds of both our past and present.

These pathological entities can either feed off the:

- earthly geopathic radiation (which is mostly spiritual), preferred by both types of demons, ahrimanic and luciferic.
- the earth's magnetic field, which is employed mainly by Ahriman, especially the ahrimanic doppelgänger.

In order to sustain their existence, however, they can only gain a foothold in the material world when they feed off the negative thoughts, actions and emotions of their host. Therefore, it is important that we gain the skills to intervene in a way that sustains a curative response towards good.

Some Definitions and Clarifications Relating to "Demons"

In this book, we will be dealing with different types of demons as discussed below:

1. Lucifer and Ahriman: These consist of highly spiritual beings, sent to assist human development by giving us the freedom of choice. However, if they become too powerful their role becomes malevolent. They accomplish this by encouraging mankind to succumb to temptation and in such a way they are able to divert us from our intended path toward divine spirituality.

2. The ahrimanic doppelgänger: This ahrimanic spirit resides in with us throughout our life. They take residence in us shortly before birth and depart just before death. We need this entity to be fully conscious in the material world. This is the ahrimanic "demon" which can be "seen" lingering in the distal, lower, part of the anatomy of both humans and domesticated animals.
3. The other doppelgängers we carry within ourselves;
    a. the luciferic doppelgänger.
    b. the karmic doppelgänger (closely related to the net of earth radiation).
    c. the "electronic" doppelgänger (a newly created etheric entity, developed by our involvement with electronic media).

    These three doppelgängers are created by our deeds and karma. The luciferic doppelgänger is the "demon" which can be "seen" lingering in the proximal, upper, part of both humans and domesticated animals.
4. The numerous smaller demons; ahrimanic or luciferic (or azuric), that are created by our malevolent actions in the past or this life. These demons can translocate when "unaware" therapists are treating symptomatically.
5. The karmic pattern that we have woven through our many lives on this planet. This weave can also hurt others.
6. "Nature"-demons created by the deeds of humans or other entities that roam in nature (Jinns as an example).

How do demons create disease?

First of all, it is important to understand that an important part of our human existence involves the presence of the two spiritual powers, Ahriman and Lucifer. Without these two entities, we would have been unable to materialize as human beings. However, when one or both of these forces become stronger than the patient it inhabits, we can through our thoughts, actions and emotions manifest pathology. In this way, the spiritual powers of Ahriman and Lucifer will cause a creation of or transformation of already existing elementals into pathological structures of demonic appearance manifesting as disease symptoms within our body.

These resulting demons gain this foothold through the actions of their host. Therefore, the causes of disease begin with the fundamental concepts of the pernicious influences of "wrong living". This can include immoral thoughts or actions, poor eating habits, alcoholism, exposure to adverse environmental conditions and other missteps in living our life. From these missteps, a deficiency develops in the etheric aspect of a fundamental process of a particular organ.[33] This weakness creates a susceptibility allowing the entrance of the demon spawned by the forces of Ahriman to not only exist but also thrive.

As normal healthy organ processes exert a check and balance over other such processes, this control is lost and luciferic demons are allowed to enter the organ process that becomes excessive as a result of such loss of restraint[34]. In other words, ahrimanic demons

---

25. The law of the five elements: a construct in acupuncture that represents a homeostatic negative feedback mechanism relating to the organ system of Chinese medicine. Each organ exerts a control over another organ to prevent hyperactivity or excessive growth (ie: cancer). In this system for example, the liver has the role of keeping check of the stomach

26. For example: the ingestion of sugar weakens the liver creating a susceptibility for the ahrimanic forces existing within the organism to act destructively on this

allow an astral access route for those that are luciferic. Over time, this excessive organ process will become also weakened, once again, allowing ahrimanic forces to thrive so that the process continues until the untimely death of the organism occurs.

Through my "spiritual eye" (clairvoyance) I have been able to actually observe the presence of these demons in diseased individuals. From my observations, I found that those with luciferic tendencies have a predilection for the upper aspect of the body, while ahrimanic demons resides in the lower aspects. In addition, I have concluded that the closer these demons are to each other (nearer to the center of the torso) the more severe is the illness of the patient. The fact is, that when they contact each other (entering the same organ), the pathology becomes extremely destructive, creating such diseases as cancer[35].

---

organ. The liver then becomes so weak it loses its ability to keep control over the stomach. This stomach yang excess now attracts a luciferic force

[35] When the ahrimanic demon 'grabs' the luciferic demon, cancer develops. When the luciferic demon 'grabs' the ahrimanic one, other destructive diseases develop, as diabetes and auto-immunity.

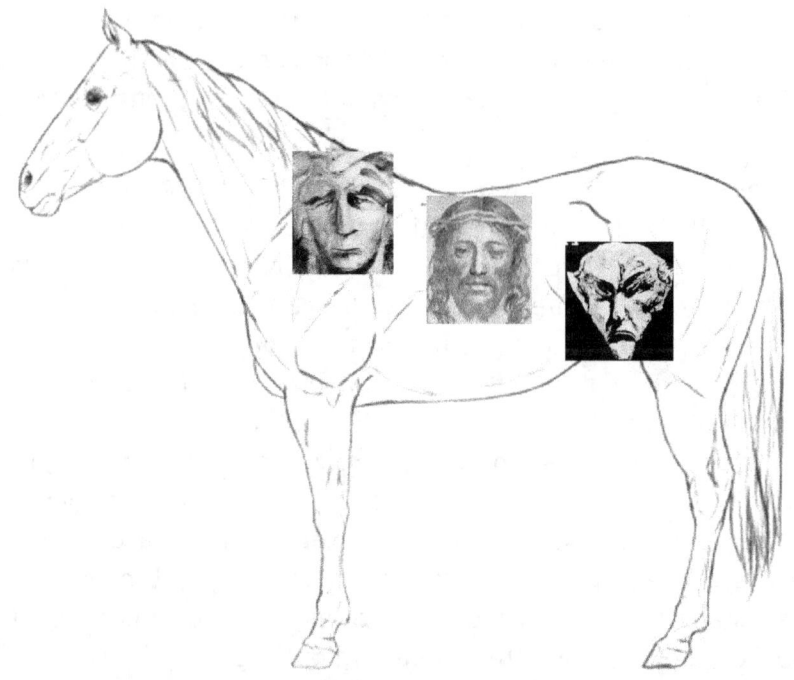

location of Luciferic and Ahrimanic demons in the body
with Christ in the middle

How do we Treat Demons? Translocation vs Transformation

The vast majority of treatment options offered patients are rarely curative due a basic ignorance of the role of these demons in perpetuating disease. For example, using typical allopathic approaches, we often subdue the excessive symptomatology (i.e.: reduce a fever). What we are actually accomplishing is a temporary weakening of the luciferic demon. If on the other hand we, as alternative practitioners, employ what we often consider a more curative approach by treating the deficiency, we accomplished only a temporary weakening of the ahrimanic demon. In circumstances when the ahrimanic and the luciferic demon join forces, as in cancer, certain drugs (ie: marijuana) that serve to strengthen the luciferic demon can appear therapeutic. This gives an edge to Lucifer, which ultimately weakens Ahriman, the more sinister of the two.

However, I have observed that the results of either treatment, serves only to drive these entities to other parts of the body, or even worse, beyond the host. In this latter situation, these demons end up "infecting" other susceptible beings. I have named this palliative approach *"translocation"*. As I will discuss in more detail in part 3, *Where Two or Three are Gathered,* I have ultimately discovered that the only path toward a cure is to *"transform"* these demons using a truly reformative process, the unconditional love of Christ. I discovered that this powerful pure energy could be unleashed by "activating" (using an acupuncture needle, or better only the fingers) a point that lies in the middle of the distance between these two entities at the region of the mid thorax. I call this point the Christ or Middle Point.

Thus, in the treatment of diseases, we are in fact dealing with five methods, of which, only the last one appears to evoke a cure:

1. Treat the overt symptoms (the excess) by subduing luciferic demons (In only 10% of these I have found that there will occur a true transformation).
2. Treat the underlying cause for the symptoms (the deficiency) by subduing ahrimanic demons. (In 60% of these cases I have found a true transformation).
3. Transforming the demons through the rehabilitative love of Christ, using the middle point (I have seen a curative transformative response in approximately 70% of my cases).
4. Transforming the demons through the rehabilitative love of Christ, using his cosmic countenance as expressed in the zodiac and his 12 apostles, using the activation of the morning-evening forces. (I have seen a curative

transformative response in approximately 90% of my cases).

5. Transforming the demons through the rehabilitative love of Christ in a group setting (see part three of this book) using the middle point. (In these cases, few of the participants (patients) respond physically curatively, but the effect here is on a deeper, spiritual level).[36]

---

[36] Please keep in mind that the curative process of the group middle treatment used by treating just the middle refers to a spiritual awakening that occurs in those ready to receive it. For the other participants, it is necessary to also apply the treatments discussed in part three relating to the pulse findings. This will be discussed in detail in later chapters

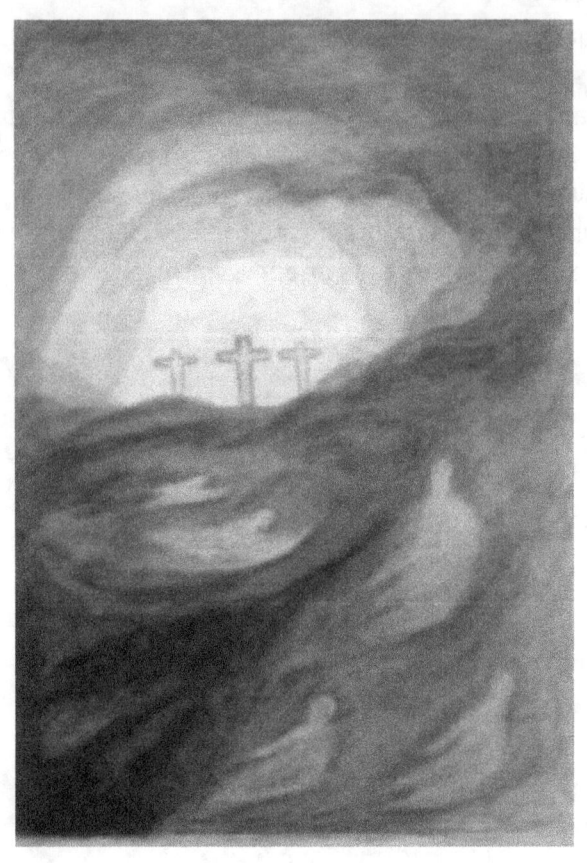

Chapter 6:

Transformation Vs Translocation

Hering's Law of Cure

As Newton asked himself why the apple fell to the ground, and thus started a whole new world of understanding, we must also ask ourselves about the real cause of the observations of what happens when we treat a patient. Within the field of classical homeopathy *"Herrings law"*[37] is a fundamental tenant which describes the direction of a curative response as healing takes place. In essence, this response is a movement away from more essential systems for survival to less important structures. For example, the asthma in a psoriatic patient will be the first condition to be resolved seen as a temporary symptom intensification while the skin pathology will be dealt with later as the patient improves. As an etheric process, these alternative modalities also work in the reverse time of this world, as healing symptoms go backward through time toward our birth. In this way, original suppressed pathologies are unearthed to be dealt with in an appropriate manner.

---

[37] Hering's law of cure: cure occurs from above to below (from the head to the limbs), from within to without (more important organs to those that are more superficial such as skin), and in reverse order of time (more recent symptoms will clear before older symptoms from the past. The disease back tracks so to speak. After the more recent problems have cleared, the patient may experience a transitory recurrence of old symptoms which soon resolve. This law is the logical inverse of the way in which chronic disease progresses with regard to the patient and the ancestral history of disease.

For me, this sort of response appears as if the symptoms are a living entity unto themselves, sometimes even leaving the body to enter the external environment. For example, after taking a homeopathic remedy, a migraine, which according to allopathic medicine might be caused by a vasoconstrictive event, appears to travel from the head outward and downward to the tips of the feet. The headache resolves and the patient may experience a return of an old toe fungus. In other words, we are treating a disease that is situated in the interior, and slowly, this ailment seems to travel more and more outward, to finally resolve with the temporary appearance of a skin lesion. Many therapists, especially homeopaths, have been trained to observe this as part of a curative process in that the vital force of the patient is expressing a healing that is going well. What has been less obvious to most healers is the possibility that the cause of these symptom reactions, may be "transposed" to other beings, whether it be a single person or a herd of sheep. A disease-causing demon in the parents may adapt to the children or their animals. I have even experienced severe diseases in patients that suddenly encompass me. One such moment occurred when I treated a migraine patient and immediately felt his throbbing pain as he began to feel improvement.

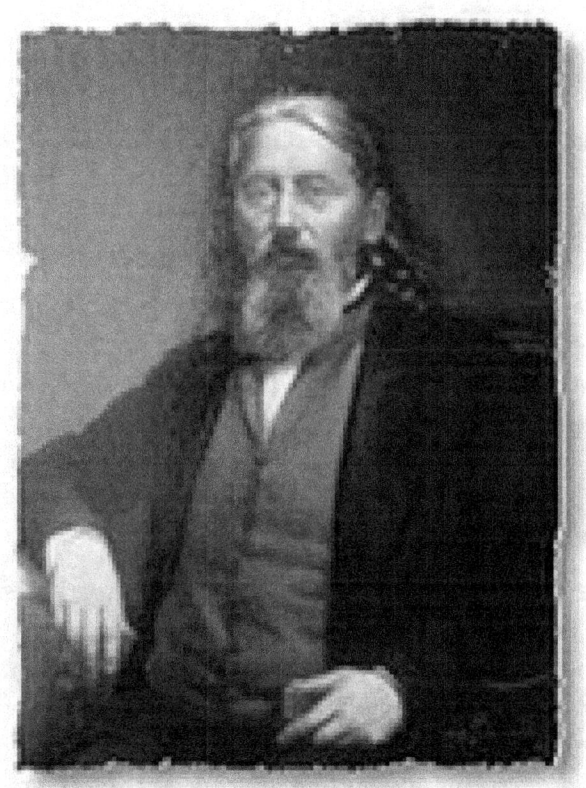

Constantine Hering
1800 - 1880

Hering's Law of Cure and Demonology: How, What and Why?

1. HOW?

For well-trained classical homeopaths, Hering's Laws of Cure are a logical part of the assessment of a patient's progress. Symptoms are always seen as a positive reaction to pathology as an attempt by the vital force to restore balance and harmony. If symptoms proceed in an outward and superficial direction, it merely shows us that the patient is improving, as they are the window to how deep or superficial a disease process has proceeded.

For a Spiritual Scientist (Anthroposophist), who acknowledges the adverse effects of demons, there is an underlying dilemma that speaks of deep spiritual disease, not only of the patient, but of all of mankind, even the cosmos. That is, how do we truly transform the patient to a higher level of health, not only for himself, but for everything that exists around him?

For me, the truth behind these symptoms relates more to the parasitizing demons or ahrimanic and luciferic doppelgängers as part of the deeper pathology. Symptoms are the footprints of the patient's pathology, but only in that the pathology is, in fact, the presence of these entities. These 'demonic footprints' are the symptoms and can be followed as they leave the patient to only invade weak and susceptible hosts that surround them.

2. WHAT?

It may now be apparent to the reader what it is that is moving from one patient to another. The answer, in my opinion, is that the symptoms my patients express are the result of the presence of a pathological entity or structure (demon). They are the wake left by the movement of this structure as it moves from the organism only to make a new home in another unsuspecting individual[38].

As discussed earlier, I have discerned the presence of two separate and distinct types of entities as being the most common pathological forces that can create disease. As with most things, these forces can have a positive influence on our development (see chapter 3 regarding elemental beings) however, in the wrong spiritual or physical environment, they can be transformed into noxious structures. It is in the infertile soil of "poor spiritual and physical lifestyles" that this change from benign entities into, what I refer to as demons, can occur.

Translocation vs Transformation

I have observed when a therapist addresses his patient, there are two common methods of treatment. Both these methods are actually a form of translocation. The first method, used widely in allopathic medicine, treats the symptoms directly. For example, one reduces a fever by giving anti-inflammatories, cooling herbs, or heat dispelling acupuncture points. I have termed this method of translocation as *treating the excess.* Or, the healer can attempt to treat at a deeper level, more commonly used in alternative medicine, by stimulating the vital force. That is, to treat the underlying fundamental weakness that created the symptoms in the first place. I have termed this as *treating the deficiency.* Earlier

---

[38] It has been my observation that internal diseases in animals can originate from their human owners or caretakers. It appears that energy goes from a greater to a lesser, whether that energy is disease or health. As such, I have found that treating the animal through its owner can yield superior results to treating the animal directly. As such, translocation always occur from a 'higher' to a 'lower' realm, or from a 'stronger' to a 'weaker' (from the astral realm to the etheric realm.

in my career as a healer, I was under the assumption that the later was the superior and more curative method. I now realize that both techniques are suboptimal, as with either modality, the pathological entity is simply transposed to another host. However, the treatment of the excess translocates 90% of the diseases, whereas the treatment of the deficiency translocates only 40 % of the diseases. It has only been in the last few years of my practice that I had come to this realization through my treatment of cancer, described in detail in the third part of this book. When my cancer treatments stopped working after 30 years of enjoying positive results, I had to question the deeper foundations of this treatment. I then knew that I had to find a method that could truly annihilate the disease.

3. WHY?

The idea of translocation implies that there is a pathological connection among all levels of creation. Within this creation there resides aspects of the spirit world that, without an inherent ability or extensive training, remain hidden to most of us. These aspects include both benevolent and malevolent beings; the latter, as I have been discussing, are referred to as demons.

Anthroposophy explains that there is a strong connection between the vast cosmos and the planet Earth, the planet Earth and its inhabitants, the inhabitants with each other and, the anatomical parts of the individual. Such complex relationships as these are the foundation of my diagnosis and treatment, whether it be anthroposophical medicine, pulse diagnosis, or treating with a group. A perfect example of this lies in the homunculi found in the individual organism. These are referred to as ECIWO systems (Embryo Containing Information Whole Organism[39]) and are a reflection of the holographic universe in which we live.

---

[39] **ECIWO** is an acronym that means **E**mbryo **C**ontaining **I**nformation of the

Spiritual Connotations of Consciousness

The old Shamans healed in the consciousness of nature. They felt connected to its forces, and the bonds that exist among all its inhabitants. As this book will reveal, the total connection to the creation leaves us also vulnerable to invasion of the malignant elementals (demons) created through our ill deeds.

Therefore, the only way for all of us to keep safe and sound is to strengthen our Spirit, in other words, our own self-consciousness. However the purpose of our spiritual evolution must not be for our own egotistical concerns (what is termed the egotistical "I") but for the purpose of all humanity (the cosmic and divine "I"). This is the only path to our salvation.

According to Anthroposophy, human evolution began in the etheric as a group consciousness. There was no thought of self, or self-identity until the appearance of Moses, who was the first person to reportedly use the phrase "I am" in reference to God. This was the beginning of our sense of self-identity. This sense of ego came to fruition with the advent of the Christ consciousness as Jesus exclaimed that he was a messenger from the "I am "and that the truth was to be found from within.

This is a philosophy, later dubbed existentialism that found fuel in the minds of 19th and 20th century philosophers. Existentialism

---

Whole **O**rganism. It indicates that all cells and parts of the body contain information of the whole body. These microsystems, such as the those found in ear may be used in therapy and in diagnosis. There are different levels of ECIWO-systems. The lowest, or primary level is the DNA-molecule. This molecule contains information on the whole organism and can give rise to all the cells in the organism. The next level is the cell, then the organ, the Organ-System and then the whole organism as such. We see this concept within botany. We may place a part of a leaf in water, and a whole new plant may arise from this. In addition, all ECIWO-systems are interconnected and by such self-maintaining and self-repairing.

spread throughout Europe, as the most important proponents such as *Gabriel Marcel, Karl Jaspers, Martin Heidegger and Jean Paul Sartre* all proclaimed that the truth lies within the "I".

Existentialism revolves around the existence of the individual as a free and responsible being who can determine his own development through the act of willing. *Søren Kierkegaard* is generally considered to be the first existentialist, believing that individuals are independent responsible, conscious beings who through their own consciousness create value and meaning in their life. His main inspiration came from the works of the Norwegian theologian by the name of *J.S. Welhaven,* who opposed the theories of extreme nationalism happening in 19th century Norway, a concept in direct opposition to the freedom of the individual. Kierkegaard's adversary was a German philosopher by the name of *Georg Hegel* who developed the concept of idealism. He believed that the fall of man was a necessary step to man's evolution. This evolution was the result of God's desire for man's complete self-awareness as inspired by Goethe.

Other historical examples of the spiritual use of the word "I", include *Mahatma Ghandi,* who during his English trial, proclaimed that the truth lies within the ability to feel the "moral inner I", *Rudolf Steiner* who stated that "Only in thinking the will, can you find the truth and the forces available for healing" and *Margit Engel* expressing that "healing is only possible if you activate your courage". In this context, the word courage implies the connection between will, intention and consciousness.

In our current time period, the idea of consciousness has been quantified using the field of quantum physics. In 1989, a physicist by the name of *Roger Penrose*, proposed that protein structures called microtubules play a role in human consciousness by exploiting quantum effects. *Thomas Nagel* is an American philosopher who postulates that each person instinctively seeks a unified worldview. He believes that a given way of understanding a subject should not be regarded as better simply for being more objective. The objective view of science when applied to the mind leaves out something essential and is fundamentally unable to help people fully understand themselves. Nagel is most widely known as an advocate of the idea that consciousness and subjective experience cannot be explained using the current concept of physics. An organism has conscious mental states only if there is something that it is like to be that organism. Others, such as *Susan Blackmore* and *Paul Churchland* argue that consciousness is a grand illusion and does not truly exist other than as an illusion of being conscious.

No matter how scientists or philosophers define it, for me, consciousness is the link to and between the spiritual beings described in this book, whether we call them elementals or demons. Through consciousness we can deal with them, and in my opinion, this is the only way to be safe in such an encounter. If we weaken our consciousness (as in the use of different drugs, such as Marijuana, LSD, DMT and so on) we are like open cups that any spirit may dive into or possess (see chapter on spirits and drugs). This consciousness reveals the hidden relationships between all living beings, humans and animals, and how therapists may cause harm through translocation to those in a relationship with the patient.

Evidence of translocation of demons by treatment

Throughout my life, my professional life in particular, I have been able to observe diseases through pulse-diagnosis and by seeing the distorted and pathological energetic structures directly with the help of my clairvoyance.

I have then observed, that after the disease has been treated; whether it be acupuncture, chiropractic, osteopathy, homeopathy or herbal medicine, the pathological structure can relocate to a different place in the body, or only temporarily be displaced to return to its original home, as a relapse in the patient's condition.

However, I would like to emphasize that diseases caused by these energetic structures may even go beyond a mere displacement within the host. These pathological entities can influence or "attack" other beings, when treated incorrectly. Therefore, this description of disease demonstrates that the symptoms display the characteristics of a separate living entity.

When studying ancient texts there are numerous examples of the concept of diseases behaving as if they are entities. I have myself experienced, as well as many of my colleagues, a sudden experience of the patient's symptoms as if a living force had entered our own interior. I have also treated patients who share the same pathology as their loved ones, as if I was treating an epidemic of a common origin, despite the fact that there is no physical evidence of a pathogen.

This speaks to the web of energy that connects all that exists in the cosmos. It lies just beyond our physical senses, to be accessible only through supra sensory perception. This "web" has been given many names whether we call it Karma, the Akashic record or even the Matrix.[40] This web is alive with the spirit world that includes etheric beings that can spontaneously arise from our thoughts and actions. We influence and effect this web every time we employ spiritual and energetic medicine.

Examples from the Bible:

In many earlier civilizations, the doors to temples of small communities were bordered by the pictures or sculptures of ugly looking demons. The purpose was to frighten the real demons or negative spirits away, in order to prevent disease. For example, there is a moving story about Jesus, told by Rudolf Steiner in his

---

[40] See the film called "The Matrix". The Akashic record: a record of all the life experiences and thought forms of a karmic nature of every human being since time began.

book *"The 5th Evangelium"*. This is a pertinent excerpt from this text regarding anecdotal evidence of disease mimicking entities:

> *"When he in his twenties visited one of the Esenic communities he then realized that the sculptures around the door scared or drove the evil Spirits away. But then a very important question arose in his mind; to where were the Spirits driven? And then he understood that it was no solution just to drive the bad Spirits away to other people, to save somebody on the cost of creating disease in others. This question and realization opened his mind to be the receiver of the Christ, the redeemer of all".*

According to Rudolf Steiner, Jesus had an epiphany regarding complete selflessness in healing an individual after observing these demonic carvings in an Esenic community. He surmised that driving spirits away was an act of disregard for the life of others as he came to the same realization that these entities could invade others. This is when he proclaimed that he must be "the redeemer of all."

Steiner again describes the same phenomenon in another book *"Spiritual Knowledge and Medicine"* from a series of 20 lectures given in Dornach from May 21 to April 9, 1920 here is a quote from lecture 2:

> *"The concept of infection, however, is none the less valid here. For any highly tuberculosis individual affects his fellow beings: and if any person is exposed to the sphere in which the tuberculosis patient lives, then it may happen that the effect turns again into a cause. I have often tried to illustrate the relationship between primary causes of a disease and infection in the following analogy. Suppose*

that I meet a friend of mine, whose relations with other people do not in general touch me. He is sad and has reason to be so, for he has lost one of his friends by death. I have no direct relationship with this friend who has died, but I become sad with him at his sad news. His sadness is, so to speak, first hand and direct; mine arises indirectly, communicated through him. Nevertheless, the fact remains that the mutual relationship between my friend and me provides the pre-condition for this "infection."

Here is another example from the above book, lecture 4:

"As individual medical men, you have the greatest interest in healing the individual patient, and modern materialistic medicine has even — one might say — sought in this way a legal justification for its aim of healing the individual. But this justification really consists in the claim that there are no diseases; there are only sick, diseased people! Now, this justification would be valid if patients were really so isolated regarding their sickness, as appears to be the case today. But in actual fact, individual patients are not so isolated. The fact that certain dispositions of disease spread over a wide region, as was mentioned yesterday by Dr. E., is of great importance. After curing one case, you can never be sure of the number of other individuals to whom you have brought the disease. The single case of disease is not viewed as part of a general process, and therefore, taken one by one, the individual result may be most striking."

Treating demonic disease with the "I" consciousness

For most disease to occur, the starting point is with some way of wrong living, thinking or feeling, or some wrong deed or karmic connection. This will weaken the etheric forces[41] of one or more of the organs of the body.

This changes the elemental etheric structure in a way that creates or invites an external pathological structure that now may be called a demon. This structure has a specific form, vibration, frequency or pattern. This entity can multiply, transform, and feed from two primary sources: Energy from the earth (referred to in anthroposophy as the nine evil layers[42]) and energy as a result of evil deeds (even if the subject perceives it is good but is covertly being used by dark cults).

Therefore, when we attempt to transform these disease-causing entities, we must consciously work with the "I" or rather with the "I am". This phrase refers to the Christ consciousness and extends far beyond the etheric level. In my earlier years, I was only treating at the etheric level using alternative modalities that achieved this goal including herbal medicine, homeopathy, and acupuncture. Although a similar and healthy version of an etheric medicinal substance or treatment could strengthen the similar etheric field of the diseased organism, this phenomenon, is also

---

[41] The Etheric body: The first or lowest layer in the "human energy field" or aura. It is said to be in immediate contact with the physical body, to sustain it and connect it with "higher" bodies. Rudolf Steiner, the founder of anthroposophy, often referred to the Etheric body ("Life Body") in association with the Etheric formative forces and the evolution of man and the cosmos. According to him, it can be perceived by a person gifted with clairvoyance as being of "peach-blossom color". Steiner considered the Etheric reality or life principle as quite distinct from the physical material reality, being intermediate between the physical world and the astral or soul world. The Etheric body maintains the physical body's form until death. At that time, it separates from the physical body and the physical reverts to natural disintegration.

[42] these being with the mineral layer and end with the earth's core. In between are layers representing qualities of extreme evil, and the fire earth connected to Natural catastrophes which are related to karma.

shared in sickness. We often see that etheric weaknesses in the owner manifest in the animal attached to him or her. This is often easy to see in regard to weaknesses shared by a dog owner and his dog. However, this communication applies to all the owner's animals whether they be cows, horses, or pigs or even the barn helpers that were hired to care for them. In essence, nervous, irritable owners will often have nervous, irritable animals; and for that matter nervous irritable employees!

Therefore, since the expression of disease is in the energetics of the etheric body, treatments are directed to change the pathology of this etheric body into a complete restoration of health. Health being defined as a curative response in all aspects of the patient. Sadly, this is often quite difficult to achieve. Due to a lack of understanding of the nature of a cure, most physicians either palliate or suppress the pathology as the patient continues to march slowly toward increasing levels of illness. From my past experience, I found that most treatments resulted in an ultimate failure to *transform* the pathological structure. It may have seemed to disappear for a short period of time (also called palliation, i.e; the return of the same symptoms unless treatment is constantly applied). Or, it may have changed, only to reappear in another more sinister form, with worsening symptomatology (suppression: the elimination of one disease state only to be replaced with a pathology that is worse than before). For example, a treatment of a cough may reappear three years later as breast cancer. This is a classic example of what is a reversal of homeopathy's Hering's law of cure. However, what homeopaths do not address in this framework, is that the disease may also travel over to another entity, whether it be human or animal. The misuse of energetic modalities can lead to confusing and varied outcomes such as the constant appearance of new symptoms, the permanent return of old symptoms, and worst of all the unexplainable appearance of similar diseases in those beings that are around the patient.

Judith von Halle gave the answer to this dilemma surrounding translocation to me during a lecture in the summer of 2013 in Berlin, Germany. She stated that the only way to transform a pathological energetic structure was to treat with the Christ consciousness; the "I am". Furthermore, she explained that it is also necessary to address the karmic cause of the patient's disease through the use of spiritual science. In this way, the therapist can use his insight, knowledge, and love to cure his patient

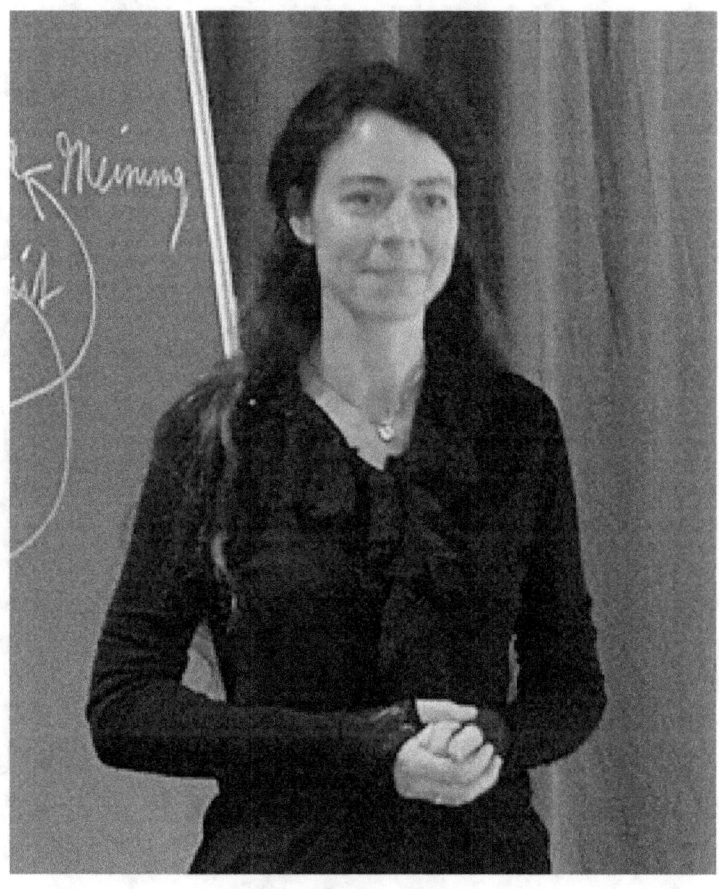

Judith von Halle

Rudolf Steiner Regarding the Concept of Shared Disease

Using the words of the Biblical Gospel according to Luke, on September 24, 1909, Rudolf Steiner lectures on the importance of the concept of shared demonic pathology among all beings and its treatment with Christ Consciousness.

> "At the time of Christ's appearance on the Earth there were many human beings in His environment in whom sins and transgressions — but especially defects of character deriving from former bad traits — were expressing themselves in disease. The sin that is actually seated in the astral body and manifests as illness, is called 'possession' in the Gospel of St. Luke. It is the condition that sets in when a man attracts alien spirits into his astral body and when his better qualities fail to give him mastery over his whole nature. In human beings in whom the old state of separation between the etheric and physical bodies still persisted, the effects of evil qualities and attributes expressed themselves conspicuously at that time in forms of illness manifesting as 'possession'. The Gospel of St. Luke tells how such people were healed through the mere proximity and the words of the Individuality now in Christ Jesus and how the evil power working in them was expelled. This is a prefiguration of conditions at the end of Earth evolution, when man's good qualities will exercise a healing influence upon all his other traits."

The above excerpt describes possession in those that suffer from the vestiges of their misdeeds, and their cure through the mere words of Christ

> "When Christ speaks of 'deeper sin' — sin which reaches into the etheric body — He uses a particular expression, clearly indicating that the spiritual factor causing the illness must first be removed. He does not immediately

> say to a paralysed man: "Stand up and walk!" but concerns Himself with the cause that is penetrating as illness into the etheric body, and says: "Thy sins are forgiven thee!" — meaning that the sin which had eaten its way right into the etheric body must first be expelled".

The above demonstrates that the cause of disease begins at the spiritual level with sin

> "In outer life itself, the effect made by one astral body upon another is quite obvious. You can, for example, wound a man by a word charged with hatred. Something then takes place in his astral body; he hears the word and suffers pain in his astral body. That is an example of mutual action between one astral body and another. Mutual action between one etheric body and another is far more deeply hidden; this involves delicate influences, which play from man to man but are never perceived today. The most deeply hidden of all are the influences, which reach the physical body, because owing to its dense materiality it conceals the working of the spiritual most completely".

The above paragraph, explains the effects of emotions on one astral body to another, and more sinister influences that are spread from one etheric body to another that can reach to the physical.

> "Christ Jesus shows that He is able to see into the very depths of the physical corporeality and to work into it. When it is a matter of working spiritually, man cannot be regarded as a being enclosed in his skin. It has often been said that our finger is wiser than we are ourselves. Our finger knows that the blood can flow through it only if the blood is circulating normally through the whole body; our finger knows that it would wither away if it were severed

> from the rest of the organism. So too, if he would understand the conditions relating to the physical body, man must know that in respect of his physical organism he belongs to humanity as a whole, that influences are continually passing from one human being to another, and that he can in no way separate his physical health as an individual from the health of the whole of humanity.

The passage above clearly plays to the fact that we all are deeply interconnected with one another and that we translocate disease to each other.

> "There came a man named Jairus, and he was a ruler of the synagogue: and he fell down at Jesus' feet, and besought him that he would come into his house: For he had one only daughter, about twelve years of age, and she lay a-dying. But as he went the people thronged him. And a woman having an issue of blood twelve years, which had spent all her living upon physicians, neither could be healed of any, came behind him, and touched the border of his garment: and immediately her issue of blood stanched." How can the twelve-year-old daughter of Jairus possibly be healed, for she is at the very point of death? This can only be understood if we know that the girl's physical illness was connected with another phenomenon in another person, and that she cannot be healed independently of that other phenomenon. When this, child, now twelve years old, was born, a certain connection existed with another personality — a connection deeply grounded in Karma. Hence, we are told that a woman, who had suffered from a certain illness for twelve years, passed behind Christ and touched the border of His garment. Why is this woman mentioned here? It is because she was connected karmically with Jairus' child! This twelve-year-old girl and the woman who had suffered for twelve years were deeply

> connected! And it is not without reason that a secret of number is indicated here: the woman with an illness suffered for twelve years approaches Jesus and is healed — and only now could He enter the house of Jairus and heal the twelve-year-old girl who was believed to be already dead."

This important chapter demonstrates Steiner's explanation of Karma's important role among us as an entire human organism, and how Christ can work through the higher "I" to heal us as a group from the ego, astral, etheric, and physical body.

> "Your Ego, in the present stage of its development, is still weak; as yet it has little mastery. But it will gradually become master of the astral body, the etheric body and the physical body, and will transform them. Before you is set the great Ideal of Christ who reveals to mankind what this mastery can mean!' It is upon truths such as these that the Gospels are founded — truths which could be recorded only by those who did not rely upon outer documents but upon the testimony of men who were 'seers' and 'servants of the word'. Conviction of what lies behind the Gospels can be acquired only by degrees. But men will gradually grasp with such intensity and strength the nature of the truths upon which the scriptures are founded that this understanding will have an effect upon all the members of the human organism."

Rudolf Steiner states that although now our higher I, our connection to the cosmos as a singular divinity is only in its rudimentary stage, it will someday develop and flourish at which time we will join him as a spiritual unity.

Chapter 7:

The Inhabitants of the Spirit World

Western Science vs Spiritual Science

Recently, I discussed the existence of demons with a Norwegian Protestant priest. I asked him the simple question, *"Does the church believe in the existence of demons"* He became irritated and replied succinctly *"We avoid this subject within the church"*. After that, the discussion came to a halt.

If we look in the gospels, there are numerous stories about demons, but the church refuses to see this. Jesus Christ and his disciples healed many people by driving away demons. A tenth of the gospels are about this phenomenon. Still, it is a taboo within the church. This is sad, but unfortunately, totally understandable.

Our western culture with its rational and materialistic viewpoint, finds the concept of non-material and invisible beings utterly irrational. The people that have started the Icelandic Elf-school or the Norwegian Angle-school are ridiculed by the sceptics and are considered by most as deranged.

However, it is my belief that this cynicism regarding the existence of a spiritual world is negative for the development of our culture and society. We have lost the reverence for both ourselves and for other beings, and consider plants, trees or animals as subordinate and devoid of a spiritual nature. Most scientists consider not even human beings as spiritual Beings. If we could consider ourselves as well as the rest of creation as part of one higher world, then we would have a much deeper respect for all life. Perhaps then we would stop damaging, killing and destroying the world as we do today. Even agriculture, animal husbandry, fishing and hunting would be employed with a new understanding regarding compassion and respect. Sadly, I have developed a pessimistic worldview. Mankind is riddled with selfishness and greed. Our only salvation is a global understanding that we are sharing this Earth with not only with each other but also a multitude of unseen spiritual beings.

We can, with our material eyes, see the plants and the animals, the trees, flowers, and insects. We feel the wind, taste the water and smell the smoke. We can immerse our physical senses in the totality of our beautiful planet. However, what our senses cannot perceive is the huge variety of spiritual beings thriving around us, imperceptible to those lacking extrasensory perception. These are qualities that are either gifts or learned skills that allow us to see into the spiritual world and its inhabitants, whether they be of an evil or pure nature.

Inhabitants of the spirit world

The inhabitants of the spirit world can be of a benevolent or malevolent nature. The prior will always be referred to as spirits and the latter, demons. The inhabitants of this world exist in a hierarchy; similar to the way the material world is organized.

1. The first hierarchy of elemental beings are the *"nature elemental beings"* inhabiting the water, air, earth and fire. They exist throughout nature and represent the spiritual basis of everything that we perceive in the material world. Even earth's crystals have spirits connected to them.
2. The second hierarchy revolves around plant life. These are group souls and are often described in folklore as Flower Fairies. In fact, every living plant and tree has an associated "fairy".
3. The third hierarchy is comprised of those spiritual beings connected with animals. Unlike flower fairies these

entities often appear unattractive to those able to see them.

4. There are also spirits that exist in the earth. These are the so-called spirits of the "earth-radiation" that create energetic grids. These grids emerge as a result of human thoughts, feeling and actions. This is the product of karma and will be discussed in detail later in this book. These spirits are bound to the people that created them as well as to the places where they were created. The part of this earth-radiation that has been created by evil deeds or thoughts may serve as "food" or "energy" for the elemental beings that are changed into vicious beings by the negative actions (karma) of humans. The variety of these geopathic spiritual beings is enormous. For example, Swedish diviners have been able to categorize more than 100 kinds of entities. Some are connected to greed, some to hate, some to murder, some to theft and so on. The ones connected to lies are the most common.

There is even a death spirit that I can spiritually see lingering behind the right shoulder of every living human. The distance between the physical body and the Death-Spirit indicates the length of remaining life of the associated being in the physical realm.

Directly attached to humans themselves, we find spirits of a higher rank than the "earth-radiation-karmic" spirits. They are mostly ahrimanic or luciferic elementals. These elementals are necessary for our wellbeing and development. However, they are capable of changing into demonic beings, depending on the level of our illness. In disease, these elementals are transformed to demons. As ahrimanic demons, they are attached to the deficient organ processes of the body. These manifest in hypo function rather than pain. luciferic demons are more attached to the psychic parts of the soul and are connected to psychiatric conditions and excessive conditions that manifest with pain.

As stated before, when observing diseased individuals, my "spiritual eye(s)" always see both the luciferic and the ahrimanic demonic spirits residing in the upper and lower aspect of the torso respectively. The further distance in the body these two spirits are from each other, the less severe the disease. The closer they are together, the more severe the disease. When they touch, or are superimposed, their destructive energy is most severe. Unless they can be separated and dissolved, luciferic and ahrimanic demons that touch each other in the body always cause destructive diseases such as cancer.

Rudolf Steiner describes that the forces of Ahriman in particular can become more destructive and predominates in today's society. It has been referred to in literature as "the double". In health, as a benign elemental, it can facilitate our wellbeing, but in illness, especially combined with a destructive life style, it can create a quite demonic structure. Oscar Wilde described the double in his book, *"The picture of Dorian Grey"*[43]. Dostoevsky also described this entity in his book, *"The Double"*[44]

In a lecture held in St. Gallen, Switzerland on November 16th, 1917 Rudolf Steiner said:

---

[43] **The Picture of Dorian Gray** is a philosophical novel by Oscar Wilde, first published complete in the July 1890 issue of Lippincott's Monthly Magazine. The magazine's editor feared the story was indecent, and without Wilde's knowledge, deleted roughly five hundred words before publication. Despite that censorship, The Picture of Dorian Gray offended the moral sensibilities of British book reviewers, some of whom said that Oscar Wilde merited prosecution for violating the laws guarding the public morality.

[44] **The Double** (Russian: Двойник, Dvoynik) is a novella written by Fyodor Dostoyevsky. It was first published on January 30, 1846 in the Fatherland Notes. It was subsequently revised and republished by Dostoevsky in 1866.

"This double about which I have spoken is nothing more or less than the creator of all physical illnesses that emerge spontaneously from within; and to know him fully is organic medicine. Illnesses that appear spontaneously from within the human being come not through outer injuries, not from the human soul, they come from this being. He is the creator of all illnesses that emerge spontaneously from within; he is the creator of all organic illnesses. A brother of his, who is not composed ahrimanic but luciferic, is the creator of all neurasthenic and neurotic illnesses, all the illnesses that are not really illnesses but only nervous illnesses, hysterical illnesses as they are described. Thus, medicine must become Spiritual in two directions, the demand for this is shown by the intrusion of views such as those of psychoanalysis and the like, where one keeps house with Spiritual entities, as it were, but with inadequate means of knowledge so that one can do nothing at all with the phenomena that will intrude more and more into human life. For certain things need to happen, things that may even be harmful in a certain direction, because the human being must be exposed to what is harmful in order to overcome it and thereby gain strength".

The spirit/soul of dead people may also hover over living humans, waiting to enter while the host is indulging in errors of living. Their alcoholic host may be drinking, a drug user is taking drugs or a sex addict is engaged in intercourse. They are like parasites and may increase the addiction and alter the host's personality.

Thankfully, there are also good spirits. Actually, all spirits are without free will, only serving their task in aiding the manifestation of the material world. It is our own actions that make them act evil. Many of the nature spirits are thus benevolent as well as many of the spirits of deceased people.

Other beneficial spirits are those of a higher-level than elementals. These include Angels and Archangels that exist to help us. However, in this same realm, there are those that are negative such as the aforementioned Lucifer and Ahriman. Not previously mentioned is a third group of potential demonic spirits named the Azuric, which represent potential disease of the future.

The Elves and Hidden People of Iceland

In the summer of 2017, I had the opportunity to visit Iceland to teach alternative medicine to a group of veterinarians as well as participate in the Elf School. It was here that we were allowed to converse with the spiritual inhabitants of Iceland. I was fortunate enough to speak with the elders of several elf tribes as well as the leaders of societies of hidden people. Our conversations were quite extensive as they told me about their history from the time of their creation as well as their hopes for their future.

The Creation Story of the Elves

This story was told to me by both the elves and the hidden people and their stories correspond on the main issues. We must first of all remember that the material existence of the human being depended on the sacrifice of both the Ahrimanic and the Luciferic realm. Without them joining human development, the incarnation of man into the physical realm would have been impossible. These, originally benign elemental forces, however, became corrupted by either dominant tendencies or egoistical desires and this stimulated both disaster and disease.

I was also told that all of the inhabitants of the sub-human realms are Ahrimanic in nature. This includes gnomes, elves, salamanders, sylfides and undines. As Ahrimanic beings, these entities can be both beneficial and potentially dangerous to mankind depending on our behavior.

The elders of one elf and two hidden people colonies then presented the story of their creation. It began with the spiritual realm, in the beginning of our existence when everything was seen as a warm etheric fluid. The cosmic plan, however, was an evolutionary path toward materialism. In order to achieve this goal, the etheric world had to develop a bipolar nature. One half of the etheric mist was to materialize while the other half was to remain[45]. In addition, these worlds became a mirror of each other, the etheric stayed upright and the material became upside down. This division is reflected in embryological development, as the fetus rotates its position in the third week of development

The order of the universe, however, favors a tri-fold existence as seen in the soul faculties of Thinking, Feeling, and Willing. This trinity is also mirrored in the world of elves. In accordance with

---

[45] 1:1: In the beginning, God created the heavens and the earth. 1:2 And the earth was waste and void; and darkness was upon the face of the deep: and the spirit of god moved upon the face of the waters. 1:3 And God said, let there be light: and there was light, 1:4 And God saw the light, that it was good: and God divided the light from the darkness. 1:5 And God called the light day and the darkness he called night, and there was evening and there was morning, one day. 1:6: And God said, let there be a firmament in the midst of the waters, and let it divide the waters from the waters. 1:7 And God made the firmament and divided the waters which were under the firmament from the waters which were above the firmament: and it was so. 1:8 And God called the firmament heaven. And there was evening and there was morning, a second day. 1:9. And God said, let the waters under the heavens be gathered together unto one place, and let the dry land appear: and it was so. 1:10 And God called the dry land Earth; and the gathering together of the waters called the seas; God saw that it was good. 1:11 And God said, Let the earth put forth grass, herbs yielding seed, and fruit trees bearing fruit after their kind, wherein is the seed thereof, upon the earth: and it was so.

these soul faculties, the elf groups are represented by the corresponding colors representing thinking, feeling and willing. The blue elves are the masters of spiritual thinking, the yellow ones of feeling, and the red ones of willing. Unlike the material world of entangled soul faculties, these elf groups work independently yet in perfect harmony, a typical attribute of spiritual inhabitants.

The Elf Cosmos.

As described above, the human realm or world is upside-down compared to the etheric realm. Although we see the elves as standing on the ground, they really touch our world with the soles of their feet. Their whole existence, consisting of cities, houses and gardens, lie within the earth, rocks and mountains. Our planet is their heaven and our cosmos is their planet or ground.

We experience this elf like cosmos after death. Our interior becomes the whole cosmos and the whole cosmos becomes our interior. That the universe is endless is an illusion of the material world. This illusion of endlessness is created by the fact that the etheric and physical cosmos are organized as a mixture of fractals as holistic constructions similar to a hall of mirrors, both in themselves and between each other. This last explanation by the elf elder was somewhat confusing as it is still a subject that lies at the edge of my comprehension.

The future of The Elves.

The elves will be trapped in the etheric world unless humans spiritualize their thinking, willing and feeling. If this doesn't happen, then these beings will remain in their etheric world and the humans in the material world. In addition, all the animals will suffer the same fate as the elves, trapped at their current level of development. This is due to the fact that the creation story of the animals is somewhat similar to that of the elves, as both share a similar splitting off from human development.

The whole cosmos is thus dependent on the spiritualization of man. For this future to be possible, Christ is helping man create a new spiritual center in the body as a new chakra. This is separate from the old system related to an upstream force paralleling the spinal cord. Nor does it relate to the chakra in front of the heart. This new chakra is just below and behind the heart and can be reached only by passing the heart and then turning back. This is the great mystery of "The turning back". The elf elder was very specific about this, he even showed me with his hands how to reach this new spiritual center of the heart

The only way to a redemption and liberation of both sides is for the material human to spiritualize so that both sides may reunite. The reunion, however, can only occur with the help of the Christ forces.

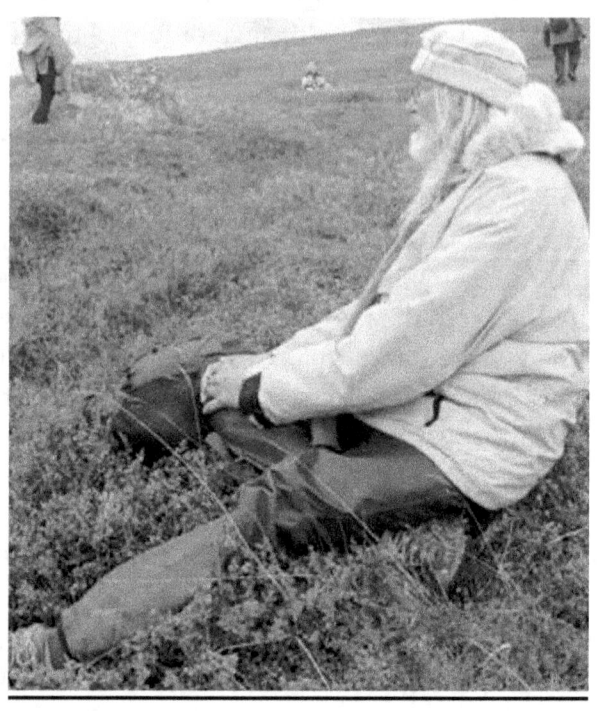

Meditating at the Elf Stone

Chapter 8:

My Personal Experiences with Demons

(much more about my encounters with demons in the book "Demons – Spiritual healing" (Temple Lodge))

The spiritual Eye

Just recently I have come to finally understand the problem of being able to "see" the spiritual world. The quotes around the word "see" are to, once again, remind the reader that this does not represent normal visual acuity. Rather, it represents the ability to perceive this world whether it is by a kind of seeing, hearing, smelling or even tasting the qualities of this alternate universe. However, I have learned that for most of my students, it tends to most often mimic the experience of seeing.

As I discussed thoroughly in part one of the trilogy, my spiritual eye was present at birth as an ability to easily excarnate from my body. I later learned that this came from my skill in separating the strong connection between thinking, feeling and willing. This is in accordance with the teachings of Rudolf Steiner, who emphasized this technique as the most important method to learn to enter the spirit world.

Another method of developing clairvoyance or the ability to excarnate can be done through mimicking a sleep-like state without losing consciousness. Normally during sleep, a division occurs between the physical body and the etheric body and the astral body and the conscious "I" function. The peculiar thing is that these innermost parts of the human being, the astral body and the ego, within which we live through (what we call soul-experience), sink down during sleep into an indefinite obscurity.

This simply means that this innermost part of the human being needs the stimulus of the external world if it is to be conscious of itself and of the material world. Hence, we can say that at the moment of falling asleep, when this stimulus ceases, man cannot develop consciousness in himself. If in the normal course of his existence, a human being was able to stimulate the inner parts of his being, to fill them with energy and inner life, then he would be conscious of them. Even when there were no sense-impressions and the sense-bound intellect was inactive and free from the stimulus of the external world, he would then be able to perceive things other than those that come through the stimulus of the senses. However paradoxical it may sound, if a man could reproduce a condition which on the one hand resembles sleep, yet is essentially different from it on the other, he could reach supra-sensible knowledge. His condition would resemble sleep in not depending on any external stimulus; however, the difference would be that he would not sink into unconsciousness and bear witness to a vivid inner life. As may be shown from spiritual-scientific experience, man can come to such a condition; a condition of clairvoyance.

Thinking, Feeling and Willing are not developed by ourselves, but are forces of the spiritual world. They are not our own abilities. They are cosmic forces.

My Personal Experiences Seeing Demons

Most of my life I have been able to see spirits and demons, creatures and entities that belong to a nonphysical world. Both can either help or cause problems for those who reside in the material world.

In the winter of 2017, I had an opportunity to spend two days in Abu-Dhabi. During that stay, I went out into the desert to experience it's desolation. I stood for a while and scanned the wide expanses of the Arabian Desert. Suddenly, a distant movement caught my attention, and caused me to focus my gaze. It soon became clear that I was looking at a group of "Jinns", the demons of the desert. Their appearance was very different from other elemental beings that I had seen before. The Norwegian elemental beings like "Nisser" and "Dverger" and even "Trolls" looked like nice schoolboys in relation to these "Jinns". They looked fierce. They sported long, sharp, tiger like teeth, and they had a very bloodthirsty look in their blood-shot eyes. I felt a certain fear as I watched them. Then one of the "Jinns", possibly their leader, caught eye of me as I was studying them. The "Jinn" realized that I saw them, and the whole group turned and rushed towards me.

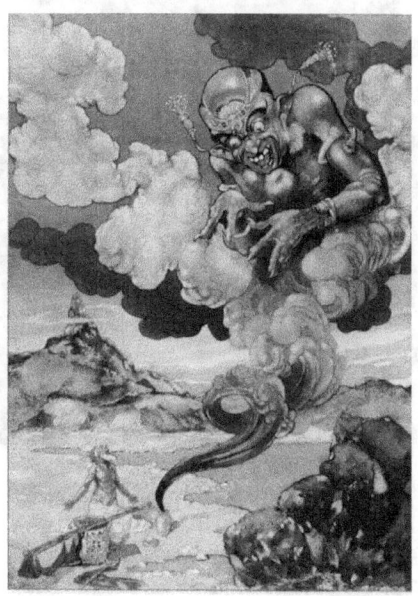

The leader of the "Jinns" stopped just in front of me and pierced me with his fierce eyes. He tried to enter me, and as I was only familiar with keeping milder elemental beings at bay, I had difficulties in keeping the "Jinn" at a distance. The strength of the

"Jinn" was overwhelming, as he pressed on towards me, and tried to get into my soul. I then remembered to make the *"Sign of Michael"*, as taught by *Rudolf Steiner*, and within seconds the "Jinn" was rendered unable to fight me. The whole group turned away and rushed further into the desert

When I later asked the local Arabs about the "Jinns", many of them had seen these creatures, and they were amazed that a white foreigner, even a Christian, had been able to see them.

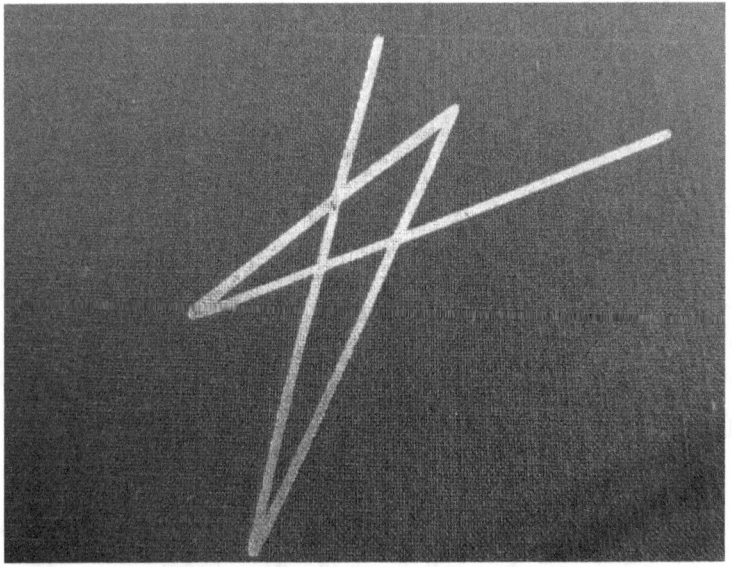

The sign of Michael

Throughout this book I will continue to ask for a suspension of judgement regarding the doubt of the existence of demons. Many will argue that they are no more than a hallucination, a product of a deranged mind. I am painfully aware that if I choose to rename these entities in a more acceptable manner, such as *"pathological structures"*, I could deflect the criticisms and avoid this discussion completely.

However, I cannot do this without lying to myself. If we seriously take what many alternative therapists, veterinarians and doctors experience, we must call them demons. As I have shown in multiple examples, these pathological structures behave like conscious entities. They move around in the body, they can jump from one being to another, and they may change behavior (demonstrated as symptoms). They may even leave, become dormant, and then return after some months. They can go back in time and display previous behaviors (return of old symptoms) or demonstrate other qualities belonging to inhabitants of the spiritual world.

As these structures do behave as if they have a conscious life, I will continue to call them Demons. In addition, I have personally seen these entities, more or less, my entire life. As I described in the introduction, I clearly visualized the date of my acupuncture teacher's death date, which proved to be accurate. This defies the physical laws of the universe and must therefore come from a spiritual sense. In addition, this ability vanished and then returned, later in my life, as an ability to see a "death entity" behind the right shoulder. The distance of the entity dictates the impending death from its host. This phenomenon of losing and gaining extrasensory perceptions is a quality found only in the spiritual world.

After graduating as a veterinarian, and moving to Northern Norway, the encounters with evil and death became more frequent. In 1980, when I was a veterinarian in the town of Bodø, a friend of my wife came to our home, complaining of a severe migraine. As soon as I entered the room where she was seated, I saw something that was partially lodged in her skull. This structure resembled a coiled snake. I then decided to take hold of this strange structure and pull it from her head. In the process of its removal, the patient proclaimed a significant reduction in her pain. I then decided to release the structure before it's complete extraction, and the woman immediately lamented that the pain had returned with a vengeance. Finally, I completed her treatment by removing the "snake" in its entirety, taking care to abolish it from the house through an open window, which later I learned to regret.

This regret emerged from the answers to a search for the many questions that I had asked myself after that fateful day. First, what was the structure? Second, where did this structure come from? And most importantly, where did it go after I released it out the window?

This search was not an easy one. I came to the realization that the journey from learning holistic medicine at a material level to the crossroads of spiritual medicine is one that must be travelled in that order. But, the precursor to starting such a journey must begin with the correct spiritual preparation of the healer. Unaware of this fact for many years, I now believe my path was always guided by the spiritual world. However, the length of time it took for me to realize this is quite humbling.

How I perceive Spiritual beings

As these beings can only be seen with the spiritual eye, I have realized that it is also important that we display a willingness to see them. When we are in the spiritual realm, we also need to "know" what to look for. Therefore, we need to not only have a strong intention and will, but also knowledge of what we are observing. If we do not know about the existence of these spiritual beings, then we will not be able to see them.

When we have become aware of and "seen" certain spiritual beings, we can build upon this knowledge the next time we use our spiritual eye. It is much like learning a skill that requires practice. Let us, for example, look at learning to play an instrument. We first learn the fundamentals, such as starting to know the placement of the fingers on the piano. The next step is learning to play the scales. Then after a while we suddenly understand the scales and are able to change between the keys.

It is in this same way that we can go further and further in seeing and understanding the contents of the spiritual world.

However, sometimes a spiritual vision is so profound that it spontaneously breaks through the veil of the material world. No preparation is necessary, and it becomes difficult to tell if we are seeing such a vision with our spiritual or physical sense organs. In addition, the more important the message brought forward by the spiritual world, the more physical the image becomes. The incident I recounted regarding the hand of Draugen was, for me, a spontaneous vision that was important enough to save my life.

Several examples of this can also be found in the Bible, when important messages of great significance for the Jewish people were proclaimed from the spiritual world. An example of this can be found in reference to the prophecies of the births of both John the Baptist and Jesus.

However, it is not only when the situation is important or dangerous for the humans involved that the perception of a spiritual being becomes very apparent, almost physical; it is also when the situation is important for the elementals or spiritual beings themselves.

Once, when walking in the forest, I came across a woman sitting beside a tree, weeping. Two men stood by her side trying to comfort her but she was inconsolable. She was weeping for the trees. I understood, after some time, that they were not real humans, but "Hulder" or "Huldra"[46], and she was being comforted

---

[46] A **Hulder** is a seductive forest creature found in Scandinavian folklore. (Her name derives from a root meaning "covered" or "secret".) In Norwegian folklore, she is known as **Huldra**. She is also known as the **Skogsrå** (forest Spirit) or **Tallemaja** (pine tree Mary) in Swedish folklore, and **Ulda** in Sámi folklore. Her name suggests that she is originally the same being as the völva **Huld**. Whereas the female hulder is almost invariably described as incredibly, seductively beautiful, the males of the same race are often said to be hideous, with grotesquely long noses.

by two "Huldre-Kalls", as described in Nordic mythology. I also tried to comfort her, but then all three disappeared. I was not supposed to see them, as this matter did not concern me. The next week huge machines came and cut down the old forest, and with that realization I almost cried.

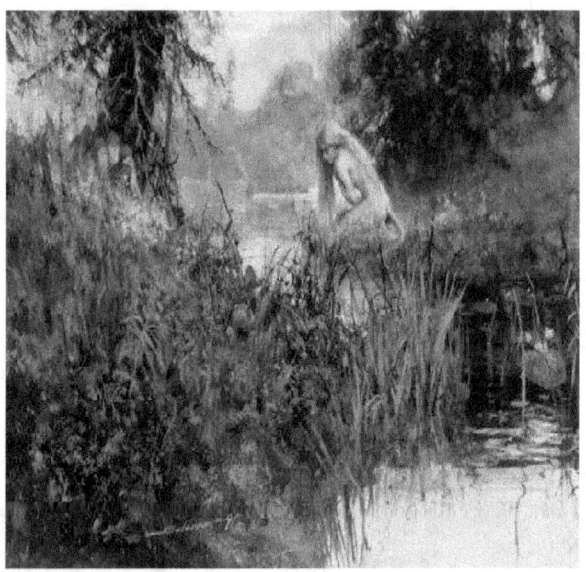

A female Hulder of Norwegian Folklore

Chapter 9:

Demons and Translocation of Disease

Most diseases in children and animals are projections from "grown-ups" especially the parents of their offspring. This is a result of translocation. This is illustrated below in a painting by Salvador Dali.

Woman, lion and horse

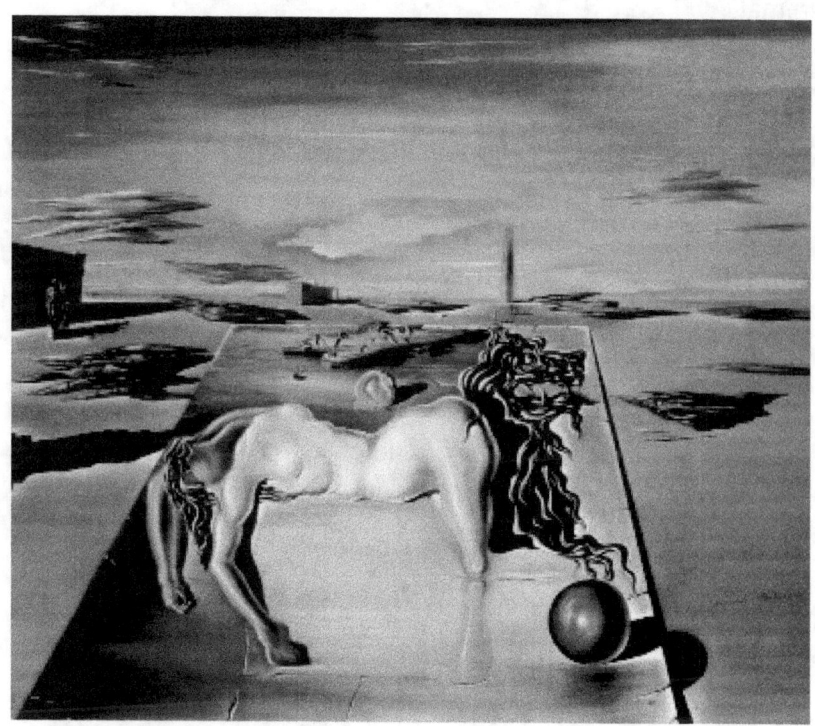

Pay attention to how Dali saw the etheric animals as being located in one direction (horse), while the astral animals are located in the other direction (lion). Between them lies the human form. It is my impression that this painting depicts both the Luciferic and the Ahrimanic being separated by man, as similarly symbolized by Steiner's statue, the "group". We can also appreciate how Dali saw man mirrored in the animal. Overall this, for me, is a truly ingenious picture.

Many animal-owners and veterinarians, including myself, have observed that their pets seem to "take on" the diseases of their owners. As a pulse diagnostician, I have verified this phenomenon by feeling that often, the pulse pattern will be exactly the same within the entire household of both family members and their animals.

Another important part of this puzzle piece came from an anthroposophical doctor lecturing at a course I attended in Czechoslovakia (Johannes Wirtzirl). He stated the following:

> "As we now know, 80% of all diseases in children originate in the parents and other closely related adults." As I listened to this statement, in my mind, I added, "and 80% of all diseases in the animals."

He then contributed another puzzle piece by also saying,

> "and furthermore, 80% of all diseases in the "grown-ups" originate from men and women not understanding each other."

In other words, Mars must come to understand Venus and vice versa.[47] I now know and understand that close to 100% of all diseases in pets come from humans.

Looking back on my veterinary practice, I now realize that for almost 40 years I have witnessed the translocation of disease from one being to another. When I accepted that 80% of all disease in both children and animals originate from the adults, I pondered the *mechanism* behind this transference of disease from man to animal and children.

I had many theories. As a medically trained physician, one may first assume it is a result of a virulent contagion. As there was often no evidence of a pathogen, I discarded this theory. Later, using my developed anthroposophical understanding of the varied sheaths of the organism, I speculated that it might be related to the etheric or astral body. This seemed to make greater sense to me as astral and etheric bodies can influence each other, as both a man and an animal.

The answer did come from Anthroposophy, but not as I had originally imagined, and I had to see it with my own eyes first to believe my conclusion. The pivotal moment came when I began to understand the role of demons in establishing disease. When I understood this, and directed my spiritual sight towards the owners and the animals, I was then able to see the demons.

Let us consider a disease such as the common flu. It spreads to (almost) all people. The pathogen carries with it an associated demon. The main demon of the disease multiplies and divides with the pathogen to infect all those that have a weakness in one of their energetic bodies (etheric, astral, "I"), through which the demon may enter. If there are no weaknesses, the person in question does not get the disease. The demon multiplies, especially if it is partially driven out by the help of allopathic remedies or symptomatic treatment (without treating the health

---

[47] Men are from Mars and women from Venus, Grey, John. Harper Collins, 1992

of the total being). After a while, it can come back to the original host, multiply and influence other members of the household.

This driving out and multiplying is described in detail in the Bible, in Matthew 12: 43-45 where it says:

> "When an unclean spirit goes out of a man, he goes through dry places, seeking rest, and finds none. Then he says, 'I will return to my house from which I came.' And when he comes, he finds it empty, swept, and put in order. Then he goes and takes with him seven other spirits even more wicked than himself, and they enter and dwell there; and the last state of that man is worse than the first. So shall it also be with this wicked generation."

Thus, Matthew describes in detail this expulsion of demons, only to have them multiply later. Another description in the Bible reads;

> 'And they came to the country of the Gerasenes, which is opposite Galilee.
>
> And when he had come to the land, there came to him a certain man from the town who had evil spirits; and for a long time, he had no clothing on, and was not living in a house but in the place of the dead.
>
> And when he saw Jesus, he gave a loud cry and went down on the earth before him and in a loud voice said, "What have I to do with you Jesus, Son of the most high God? Do not be cruel to me"?
>
> For he gave an order to the evil spirit to come out of the man. For frequently it would take a grip of him: and he was kept under control, and prisoned with chains; but parting the chains in two, he would be sent by the driving of the evil spirit into waste places.

And Jesus said to him, "What is your name"? And he said, "Legion"; for a number of spirits had gone into him.

And they made a request to him that he would not give them an order to go away into the deep.

Now there was a great herd of pigs in that place, getting food on the mountain: and the evil spirits made a request to him that he would let them go into the pigs, and he let them.

And the evil spirits came out of the man and went into the pigs: and the herd went rushing down a sharp slope into the water and came to destruction.

And when the men who took care of them saw what had come about, they went quickly and gave news of it in the town and the country.

And they went out to see what had taken place, and they came to Jesus and saw the man out of whom the evil spirits had gone, seated, clothed and with full use of his senses, at the feet of Jesus; and fear came on them.

And those who had seen it gave them an account of how the man who had the evil spirits was made well.

And all the people of the country of the Gerasenes made a request to him to go away from them; for they were in great fear: and he got into a boat and went back.

But the man from whom the evil spirits had gone out had a great desire to be with him, but he sent him away, saying,

Go back to your house and let them have news of all the great things, which God has done for you. And he went away, giving word through all the town of the great things which Jesus had done for him".

(Luke 8: 27-40)

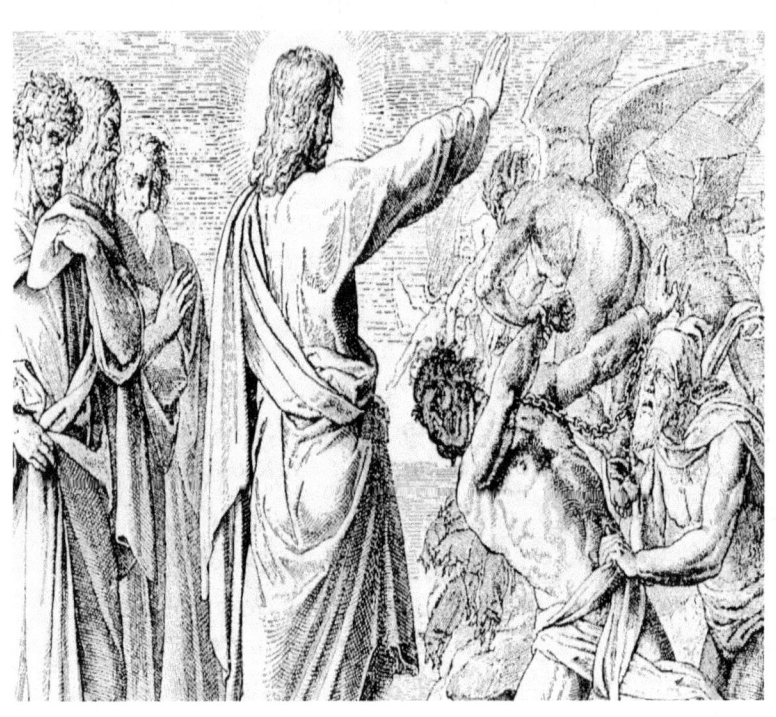

More on Ahriman, Lucifer and Azuras

1. Ahriman

When ahrimanic demons enter or are created in the body, the results are always negative. How they affect us depends on our personal weak areas (susceptibility). If, for example, they enter into *the physical body* we become physically ill. This can manifest as poor circulation, sclerosis, and exhaustion. If they enter into *the soul* we may become uncompassionate, selfish and narcissistic. If they enter into *the spirit,* we become ignorant towards the spiritual world, atheistic, hostile and in denial towards religious beliefs. The influence of Ahriman surrounds us as we fall prey to the worship of money reflected in a society devoid of empathy and ultimately invested in profit motive.

2. Lucifer

When *luciferic demons* enter us, the affect is a disinterest for the material world. We become over occupied with the occult and are easily drawn into cultish behaviors that mimic spiritual enlightenment. If the susceptibility is in our physical body, we can develop painful and febrile inflammatory conditions, such as infections and autoimmune disease. If the soul is weak, we become bound up with negative emotions such as greed, jealousy or anger. We can often develop delusions of grandeur and a type of specialness prevails, with exaggerated perceptions of our importance. If Lucifer finds a pathway into the spirit, we become confused, depressed and misled on our spiritual path. We have the tendency to believe in all kinds of spiritual movements. This can be seen very clearly in India where large populations are dedicated to the worship of the old Luciferic oriented gods (gods who became irrelevant after the advent of the Christ consciousness). In India, there is little concern for the immediate surroundings relating to garbage, air pollution, and the suffering of animals, children and women. Luciferic demons cause us to become obsessed. For example, some become maniacally artistic, producing art that has nothing to do with reality. Egotistical and self-occupied, these luciferic types are often diagnosed with bipolar disorder and addictive tendencies.

3. Azuras

Another class of demons are termed the *azuric demons*. These demons, cause us to lose our higher self (I consciousness) leaving us disconnected from the cosmos, and as such, we become self-centered and easily influenced by Ahrimanic knowledge. This knowledge will ultimately inhibit our human evolution.

Demon Prevention

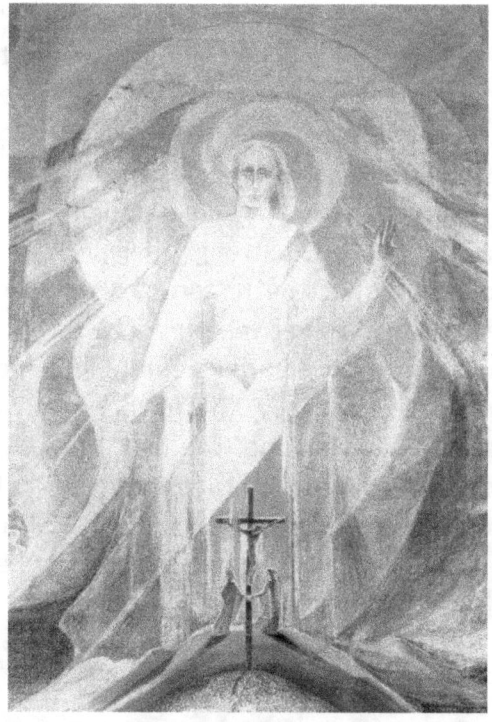

A logical question to ask at this point is, how do we protect ourselves from demons? What I have learned so far are two important concepts.

We must learn to develop a strong self-consciousness also called the "I AM".

The consciousness of the "I AM"

This represents the light that leads us out of error and corruption and enables us to find our way past both the ahrimanic and the luciferic demons. The beginning of the material world began when the "I" descended from the spiritual world and became ensnared by desires and cravings. This was facilitated first by Lucifer, and then, additionally enslaved by Ahriman's influence. As a result, man became lost in the earthly, physical world of lies, error and illusion. This is when man lost his direct connection to the spiritual realm. He lost the understanding of the Spiritual world and how it operates. I strongly believe that this Spiritual connection somehow must be restored. If not, we will forever become slaves, trapped under the influence of both Lucifer and Ahriman. Transformed adversarial elementals can enter man on many different levels. Basically, the further into the body they reach, the more damage is done. The first "step" is an attack on the Astral body, or less often, on the Etheric body. The next step is the Etheric body, and the last step is the physical body, although some theorize that the "I" is the last and most dangerous step.

Chapter 10:

Earth Radiation and Karma: Demon Food

Karmic demons

Demons can be divided in two groups according to when and how they are created. The first group contains the demons created by human actions and the second, demons existing from earlier cosmic development. I find it extremely difficult to make a differentiation between these two groups, as they appear quite equal, although I know that they are on many levels, different.

Demons are always involved in the development of disease, both in animals and in man. Concerning diseases in humans relating to both the body and the soul, the most significant demons are those we have created through our deeds, thoughts and feelings. They are referred to as "karmic" demons.

I was visiting a friend of mine who suffered from episodes of severe depression. His moods during these moments was so debilitating that he could not work for weeks or months. He had no idea why he would become so depressed. At the time I was visiting him, he was not experiencing his spell. I sat at the table, and he went to the kitchen to make me an espresso. Suddenly, he sank into a dark mood. I could see the cause of his depression. A huge dark Demon began to engulf him. I tried to ask the Demon why it came, but it would not answer. I continued to ask the entity how old it was, and finally it responded that it had been created by a dark action committed by my friend's grandfather. The action had to do with an act of immorality.

I told my friend that he must search for the nature of this immoral act and then ask for forgiveness for his grandfather. I found that if this is properly performed, the demon will disperse and vanish, having been freed and transformed. We must not just push the Demon away, as it desires transformation.

Demons and "Earth-radiation

Demons can also be created by the presence of a form of radiation that emerges from the Earth. This particular etheric force is a central concept in the development of my understanding of the role of demons and the way in which they create disease.

Since 1972 I have been investigating, what I refer to as, ley-lines that form a grid of *"Earth-Radiation"*. Since 2004 I have been able to actually *see* this matrix of energy[48]. These ley-lines are not measurable with physical devices and, as such, I realized I was aware of such energy through the use of my *"spiritual eye"*. Therefore, these grids are of a spiritual origin.

This "spiritual radiation" should not be confused with the grid of electromagnetic energy that causes disease in living beings, as what is emitted from high-voltage installations and cell phones. This *Spiritual Energy* is a combination of the emanation from the demonic layers of the earth and the expression of the ahrimanic entities created by human misdeeds from the past. This "Spiritual Substance" is thus both the demonic entities themselves and a kind of fuel or food for the ahrimanic entities, including "The Double. This emanation therefore, fuels the karmic demons and causes disease. This is especially true if one sleeps over such radiation or is connected to it.

There are those that are capable of discerning these grids with the help of kinesiology, using divining rods or pendulums. They are often hired by patients to determine if this sort of etheric radiation

---

[48] Described in my book "Holistic Veterinary Medicine" published on Amazon. It can also be obtained in Norwegian, Swedish, Spanish, German and Italian. Also described in my book "Poplar", published on Amazon, which can also be obtained in Norwegian (Poppel) and German (Pappel).

could be the cause of their pathology. After discovering the presence of the noxious radiation, methods such as copper threads and other devices are used to alter the ley-lines. Although they are able to ameliorate the condition, the radiation returns requiring monthly treatments to keep the radiation at bay.

I have evaluated the work and efficacy of many who work in this field of "diverting" Spiritual earth-radiation. My conclusion from these observations is that this matrix or grid of Earth-Radiation is not only changeable, but alive having an intention of its own.

I later discovered that these lines of Earth-Radiation not only changed, but moved several meters by themselves, especially if someone tried to alter, disperse or stop them. Furthermore, I made the astonishing discovery that I could move them by my own will and Intent. I started to demonstrate my ability to dowsers. During a course, I moved a "lay-line" through the room so fast that many of the participants felt it like a soft wind that swept through the area. I can manipulate the earth-radiation because of my ability to "see" them.[49] After seeing the energy, I then fixate on them with my will power and move them to another location.

I have used this method several times. During a Veterinary Acupuncture Course in Germany, the leader of the German Dowsers Association was demonstrating how to find "Earth-Radiation Lines". She had dowsed an area of the forest beforehand and had found radiation lines there. Her task was to show the class how to find them and mark them with coloured paper.

---

[49] **Earth-Radiation** is "seen" (at least I see it this way) as snakes traversing the room, or the forest. Black and shiny, going from left to right or from right to left. One direction goes from the past to the future, and the other direction goes from the future to the past. At a certain level this energy has the shape of a snake, on a higher level it has the shape of a Demon. Before 2014 I saw the Demons in the shape of snakes, and mainly as "earth-radiation". Lately I can see them as Demons, clinging to humans, causing diseases and pain, depressions or anger. Even Death can be seen in this way.

I stood, watching from a distance. Just before she was ready to demonstrate the presence and effect of the lines to the group, I moved all the lines to another place. Then I waited for the results. She started to look for the lines, but she could not find them. She became very frustrated. This was when I realized that my vision and actions were objective. This led me to understand that the "Earth-Radiation lines" are living entities that can be manipulated by my soul faculty of willing, which infers they are absolutely Spiritual in origin.

For years I investigated these grid lines, which appeared as "black snakes". A peculiar quality I discovered about these oscillating structures was that they opened my spiritual senses to time itself. They did not only stream between trees and other living entities, but they also streamed between past and present, and between present and the future. I discovered that I could also travel inside them to the past (always towards the left) or into the future (always to the right), with the latter, I seldom dared to try. If we do not enter the "snakes" deeply but stay in the periphery, the directions of time are opposite.

I heard that, in order to travel out-of-body in time and space, Shamans of indigenous cultures project their Spirit into "Benevolent Spirit Guides". Apparently the "Black Snakes" represent my Guides. When I travel within them, it really seems as if the past or the future is coming toward me. When the past comes into my consciousness, it is like an encounter with an ahrimanic demon or Spirit. When the future comes into my consciousness, it is like an encounter with a luciferic demon or Spirit, but as I stated previously, I seldom dare to travel to the future.

When my consciousness encounters these two Time Streams, one from the past and one from the future, I face The Double Stream of Time. This is a very important and hidden mystery. I will not discuss it further in this book, except to say that it can be met within the Elemental World of the Trees. When I travel inside these streams into the past, I experience strange and changing plant-forms that have not been seen for millions of years. With this travelling technique, I can investigate the leaf forms as long back as ancient Silurian times.[50]

Once, I totally lost myself when travelling back in time. I can usually step out of the described "streaming black snakes" easily, but this one time it was impossible. I disappeared into the past. I opened my physical eyes, but still I could not see the present. I was really in the past. I saw, with open eyes, the dinosaurs walking past me just as if I was actually there (which I believe I really was). I saw the old forms of trees and plants growing around me and I was taken further and further back in time. I started to become frightened. I tried several methods to come back to the present time but was totally unable to do so. After a long while I managed to come back using old Shamanistic rituals to help me.

I now understand how these grids or matrix of "snakes" were created. They are created by the evil or egoistic deeds of humans and fed by the upward streaming forces of the deeper layers of the earth. If the human being that created the elemental demon is dead, the grid-line remains. In this period it may cause disease or discomfort in other humans or animals that happen to sleep or live where the lines are located. In a later life, when the maker of the line is reincarnated, the spirit of this reincarnated human is drawn to the site where the line awaits. When he or she then comes again to the area of past sin, the grid-lines (demons) attach to the human who then remembers the past deeds. Ironically, the perpetrator always returns to the scene of the crime.

These lines are made up of elementals if they are benevolent, or demons if they are malevolent. These malevolent grids are the ones connected to our karma. If their makers are in the otherworld, the demons may haunt other people while they wait

---

[50] The **Silurian time** is a geologic period and system that extends from the end of the Ordovician Period, at 443.8 million years ago (Mya), to the beginning of the Devonian Period, 419.2 Mya.

for their "makers" to be re-born. Thus, these lines or grids contain the entire history of our lives as the *"Akashic Chronicle"*. Karma and the Akashic Chronicle are interwoven in these lines, and as such are two parts or realities of the same grid.

The entire world is full of these demonic grids, fed by the upward streaming of Ahrimanic forces from the depths of the Earth. They are of many kinds and appearances. Some are made by greed, some from anger, murder, violence, and jealousy and others from pain or sorrow.

In the Old Norse book *"Edda"*[51] a similar phenomenon is described, relating to the *"Nornes"*[52]. The Old Vikings *"saw"* that when a child was born, a *"web"* was waiting for it. Three women were waiting to connect the child to this web, which represented the karma of the infant. The names of the three women were past, present and future (Vilje, Verdande and Ve, or also called Urðr (Wyrd), Verðandi and Skuld). The "Nornes" also had a scissor to cut the thread when the task of this life was fulfilled. This description for me is an accurate description of the web that I observe, the cause of its existence, and how it is created.

---

[51] The term **"Edda"** (/ˈɛdə/; Old Norse Edda, plural Eddur) applies to the Old Norse Edda and has been adapted to fit the collection of poems known as the Poetic Edda. Both works were written down in Iceland although they contain material reaching into the Viking Age. The books are the main sources of medieval tradition in Iceland and Norse mythology

[52] The **Norns** (Old Norse: norn, plural: nornir) in Norse mythology are female beings that rule the destiny of gods and men. The three most important norns, Urðr (Wyrd), Verðandi and Skuld, come out from a hall standing at the Well of Urðr (well of fate).

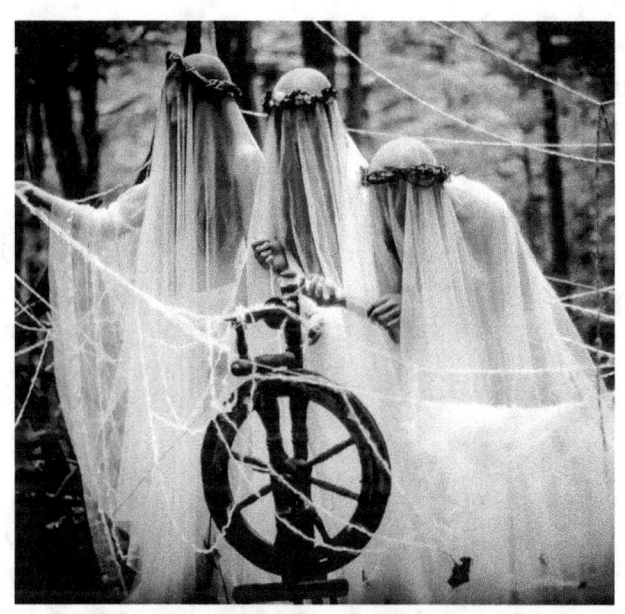

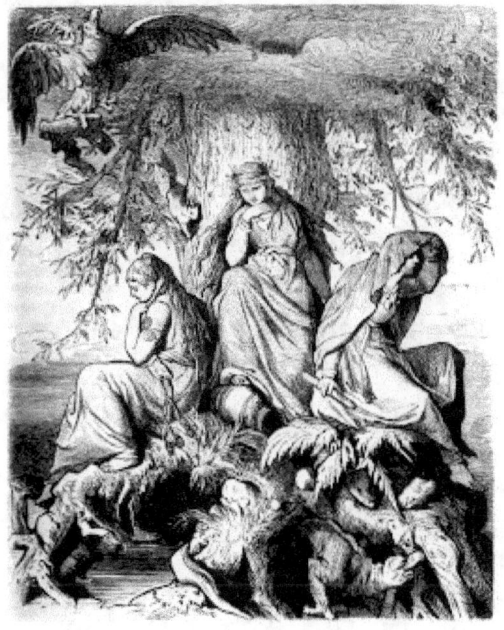

The Nornes of the Nordic mythology

When I started to understand this, the connections between "Earth-Radiation" and man became clearer. I saw how the actions of man created or attracted the snakes/demons, and how these Demons created diseases and disasters in man.

Such demons may also create disease in people that live close by or are attached to those who carry these entities. Over the ages, it has been observed that living or sleeping on earth-radiation may cause disease as a demonic possession and that freeing oneself of such an affliction is impossible unless one learns the way. (See part 3, *Where two or three are gathered*).

Demons can also be created through deeds of violence towards nature. If we cut down a tree, if we kill weeds or insects by the help of chemicals (Roundup), if we slaughter a healthy cow or horse, or if we cut down whole areas of forest with huge machines, strong disharmonic demons will be created.

Summary of the action that create demons

- All our actions through passion, such as greed, hate, jealousy and anger create luciferic demons.
- All deeds done with the help of machines, cold thoughts, slaughterhouses or cutting down trees create ahrimanic demons.
- All deeds that betray the truth, lead people astray or convert religions create Azuric demons.
- Demons of a lower rank than humans, especially those of the 3 elemental regions, are created by man.

Summary of Earth-Radiation
1. Radiation from the earth, mainly of Ahrimanic influence.
2. Electromagnetic radiation created by human technology (high voltage pylons or mobile phones, influence both ahrimanic and luciferic demons).
3. Spiritual radiation from actions committed on the spot where the radiation is found (usually called "Geopathic Radiation") is caused mainly by ahrimanic demons. They have a huge influence in the creation of disease.
4. Spiritual radiation (both luciferic and ahrimanic Demons) that follow the single human being. They cause disease mainly for the person in question, and work through both the ahrimanic and the luciferic doppelgängers.
5. Radiation from the cosmos (from higher beings of many kinds, among other demonic, Angelic or planetary beings).

The relationship between Earth Radiation, Karma, demons, disease and the Moon[53]

Steiner lectured extensively about Karmic relationships and in several of these lectures he discussed the effects of Earth Radiation on this subject. Written below are pertinent excerpts from these enlightening lectures:

> *The Moon and the Sun (1/25,1924): The moon and the sun are the two gates through which the life of man in its*

---

[53] Rudolf Steiner in 1924 gave a series of 84 lectures regarding Karma. The resolution of individual karma is essential to the spiritual evolution of all of mankind and must be understood in the context of the history and future of cosmic evolution. In Steiner's cosmos, seen with his spiritual eye he perceives the cosmos and the evolution of humans as a co-joined event broken up into phases that are reflected in planetary stages. More on this in the final chapter of the trilogy.

totality reaches beyond the physical world. The Moon endows us with individuality, representing the past. The Sun gives access to the universal human representing the future. This is necessity verses freedom. In the destiny of two individuals, the Moon and Sun existence are at work: The connection before the meeting Is determined by the Moon Existence, by necessity; happenings after the meeting is determined by the sun, by freedom. After the Karmic meeting of two human beings the thread of the karma reaching far back into the past is woven into the thread stretching into the future. New faculties of perception bring knowledge of cosmic destiny. The esoteric conception of necessity and freedom.

Beings in the heavenly bodies (1/28/ 1924): The moon beings keep the records of past humanity and of every individual man. Such records determine karma. This is the function of the Angeloi in cataloging the differences in the meetings of individuals. These are the links between an Initiate and those with whom he comes in to contact. These records also contain the characteristics of the biographies of initiates.

The two portals into the spiritual world (2/06/1924): The primordial wisdom on Earth was imparted by lofty spiritual beings who went to the moon after it separated from Earth. These beings record the destinies which individuals have in common. They are also in charge of the change and replacement of physical substance in heavenly bodies as well as in man.

We have seen that the web that the Nornes have been preparing for each individual is somewhat related to the earth through the ground upon which the individual is living. This karmic energy can influence others living in the same area, or even more so, if they are sleeping next to one another. The memory contained in the etheric body will additionally mingle and become similar if they also engage in sex. This web is deeply related to the moon.

In 1984, I befriended a couple whose occupation was to form a protective barrier against earth radiation for their clients' homes. At that time, I was unaware of the foundation of this type of radiation. The more sensitive woman served the role of radiation detector while the man constructed radiation resistant copper wire around the noxious area.

However, I discovered, through my spiritual eye, that the copper wire failed to instill protection after the appearance of the next full moon. As an experiment, I asked the couple to examine my basement in which was found a very strong lay-line. I then handed her a picture of the full moon concealed it in an envelope. I then asked her, while holding the envelope, to dowse for the radiation.

Shockingly, as she passed along the lay-line, some unseen force wrenched the rod from her hands, smashing it against the wall. The woman then proceeded to faint, falling to the floor. After she awoke they left abruptly never to return.

Why are only some people influenced by such earth-radiation and others are especially resistant? I have discovered through clairvoyance, that these sensitive people have areas of openness in their aura. Furthermore, I surmised that this susceptibility is karmic in its origin and in these particular cases, closely related to the moon. I have postulated that the effect of the moon has to do with at what point in their spiritual development their Karma was forged.

For those who are not easily influence by the moon, have had their Karma forged at a different point of their spiritual development (sun). These people have detached themselves from the earth as well as their national spirit. Such people are referred to by Steiner as the homeless, seen as high-level initiates who are able to identify themselves with the great mission of humanity as a whole, without the particular feelings for a certain nationality.

Therefore, in this case homelessness is actually a detour to higher spiritual development only to finally return as leaders of these groups to further evolve mankind. This is so that these individual folk groups can bring the knowledge of their folk souls to the common spiritual evolution of mankind.

The history of obvious and detectable effects of the "earth-radiation".

Radiation from the earth and from aquifers (natural water lines in underground rock fissures) has a long tradition. One early reference is found in the books of Moses. The story tells of the Israelites thirsting in the desert. Moses took his stick and hit the rock, and out gushed water. The German expression "Rotenschläger" (to hit or beat something with a rod) refers to the European tradition of diviners using twigs or Y-sticks from hazel or other trees to locate water or metals underground.

There are many references of such events throughout history. It is mentioned in China that emperor Kuanggu (2400 BC) made laws about how land used for building houses should be examined beforehand in relation to Geopathic Radiation. Fengshui Yingli is the Chinese term for Geopathic Stress. It literally means Wind and Water Stress. The Chinese system of Fengshui includes an examination of the area for Geopathic Lines. These are called Dragon Paths (Longlu), or Dragon Channels / Vessels (Longmai). The geopathic Demons cooperate in strengthening the disease created by the Demons abiding in the body of the person that sleeps there. Fengshui is still used today to position doors, windows, rooms, mirrors, beds, work areas, wind-chimes, etc in the interiors of houses, shops or hotels etc. Its aim is to get the best flow of Natural Energy throughout the building and to banish, or avoid Geopathic Energies where possible.

Several Indian cultures in North America share the same concepts. If a tent was to be put up, or a camp built, one must first sit down and talk with the Spirits about whether it was the right place or not. This practice can be found especially among the Hopi Indians in America. In India, we find the same tradition where it is of great importance to find the right place for a bed to be placed. Several woodcarvings from 14th-16th century show diviners (branch-bearers) searching for earth-radiation of various kinds.

Illustration of "dowsers" from 1494.

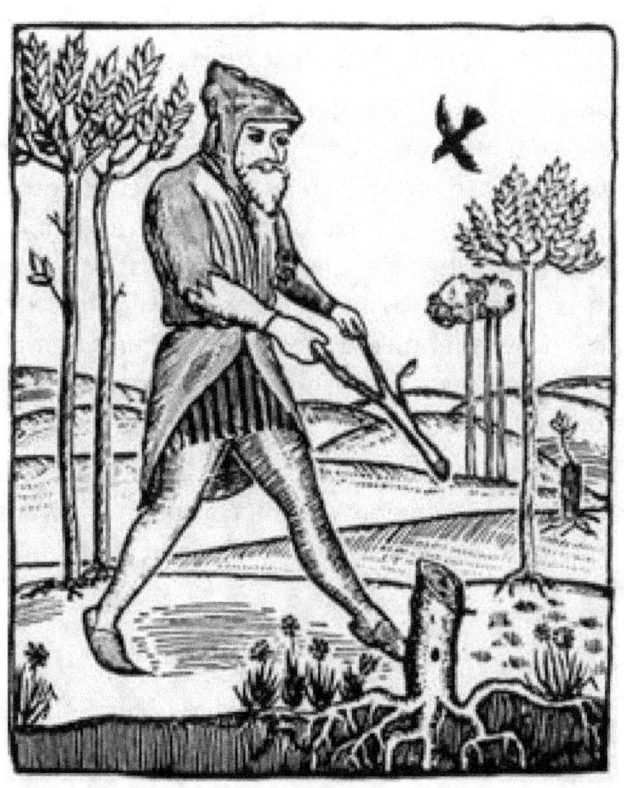

The Earth's Physical Electromagnetic Fields

Applying the physical research of electromagnetic radiation to my spiritual work on demons, I have concluded that the electromagnetic field of the earth itself is related to the cooperation of Ahrimanic and Luciferic demons. Ahriman in my opinion, appears to thrive on electricity while Lucifer has an affinity for magnetism. As such, the ahrimanic forces works through the electric phenomena of the nervous system, while the luciferic doppelgänger works through the static fields of the circulatory system, related to the blood-vessels as described by the Swedish scientist Björn Nordenström[54].

Over millions of years, our biorhythms have developed and become dependent on the earth's fluctuating electromagnetic fields. We are in fact dependent on the existence of both Ahriman and Lucifer to develop as human beings in full freedom. However, Illness occurs both when the physical Earth-Radiation, especially that which is produced by man, is too strong. As a result, the appearance of degenerative diseases will occur when ahrimanic demons are the strongest, and infectious diseases escalate in the presence of Lucifer.

Environmental Earth-Radiation includes electric fields, radio, TV, laptops, computers, equipment that uses microwaves, high frequency radiation such as alpha-, beta- and gamma- radiation,

---

54

During the 1950's, a Swedish radiologist and , Dr. Björn E.W. Nordenström became interested in streaks, spikes and coronas that he saw in X-ray images of lung tumors. When he discussed his observations with other physicians, many of his colleagues saw nothing. Others attributed the phenomena to artifacts in the image. In 1965 Nordenstrom began an investigation on these anomalies and theorized a closed electrical loop circulatory self-regulating model for healing. He used this concept to create a unique electrochemical therapy that supports the natural endogenous current that supports healing

Cosmic Radiation and other Geopathic Radiation. All these forms of radiation affect us. We meet these influences in our everyday life as sound, light and other electromagnetic and spiritual radiation. Our senses normally do not perceive such forms of radiation, but dowsing can.

All these forms of Earth-Radiation interfere with each other. They create complicated patterns that influence the organs of the body, as well as their processes and biorhythms. The influence of this radiation varies from one individual to the next and from one place to another. That is why it is difficult to predict which human or animal will develop disorders, which places will manifest the disorders, or which specific disorders will arise from these influences. However, despite this, it is very important that we can diagnose the cause.

In my opinion, two of the most important factors in developing disease from the influence of Earth-Radiation are the strength and virulence of the demons behind the electric, magnetic or spiritual radiation present at any given site, and the vulnerability of the three auras that surround us; the Etheric, Astral and I Consciousness aura. Many people who are especially sensitive to earth-radiation have "holes" in their auras, through which the Demonic Influences may enter and leave.

I have observed that almost all people who are hypersensitive to earth-radiation have distinct holes in their Aura, which must be closed if they should have any chance of regaining normal health. This closure may be brought about mainly through understanding the cause of the hole, which may be a former trauma, misuse of drugs or immoral/wrong thought-forms, but also by physical means such as wrappings of wool or turf.

As Dr. Becker[55] concludes, it is important not to disturb normal Earth-Radiation and magnetic fields and, in so far as is possible, to limit man-made and artificial fields, or excessive natural fields. We should avoid strong artificial radiation from mobile telephones, high-voltage cables, transformers and electric equipment. We should also avoid strong Geopathic Radiation, especially that over crossing aquifers or those relating to earlier misdeeds carried out on that particular spot.

We should also try to develop our ability to detect these stimuli (or get help from others to do so). And finally, we should educate as many people as possible of the existence of these noxious effects.

---

[55] **Dr. Robert Becker**, a US Army surgeon i wrote the best explanation of this theory in "The Body Electric," His book describes 30 years of his research on the importance of effects of the body's electrical signalling system.

Becker concluded that electrical currents exist within the body as a form of slow acting "Primitive Nervous System," analogous to that of plants and invertebrate forms of animal life. This system uses a cell-to-cell signalling by direct electrical currents to control many of the body's slower-acting processes, such as those of wound-healing, tissue regeneration and growth.

Becker became interested in bioelectricity as part of his research on tissue regeneration in US soldiers that were badly wounded in battle in the Far East. While amputating salamander tails, he discovered that a special electric pattern arose before the amputated tail was fully regenerated. Frogs, who do not have the ability to regenerate amputated limbs, show a totally different electrical pattern. He hoped that this could lead him to a solution as to why various bone fractures do not knit again. He concluded that bone fracture healing in all types of organisms depend on the electrical pattern, much resembling his observation of salamander regeneration.

Effects of Geopathic Radiation.

On Plants.

Effects of geopathic stress on plants include twisted growth in plants and dead or stunted gaps in the avenues of trees. Fruit trees are most sensitive; while redwoods and ash are the most resilient. Garden hedges can show the effects of geopathic radiation clearly as some hedge-shrubs under the influence of this radiation, die or become stunted. These affected shrubs have fewer and smaller leaves. Similarly, the hedges do not look healthy and appear uneven, often seen with a variety of significant gaps.

The first reports of the effect of geopathic radiation on plants came from Germany in the late 1800s. Fruit trees, especially apple trees, tend to grow away from the geopathic radiation. They become crooked, deformed and non-productive. Some trunks split in two and the branches that grew directly over the area of radiation became deformed. Cherry and sweet cherry trees demonstrate stunted development, malformed branches and cankers, the latter, often effecting birch trees. In fact, cankers on birch trees are quite common in areas of geopathic stress, where whole groups of this tree present with the characteristic "crow's nest" of canker. Although it is shown that viruses cause these tumors, it does not explain why some trees are attacked and others are not. It is the same as in humans and animals; viruses and bacteria surround us, but disease can manifest only under certain conditions. For example, stress can weaken the immune system of plants and animals, allowing bacteria, viruses, fungal infections to thrive. Therefore, it is of utmost importance to appreciate that disease is not a direct result of external pathogens, but more due to the susceptibility of the host. Unlocked homes invite thieves.

Immunosuppression is a common form of susceptibility and can be induced by exposure to excessive Earth-Radiation over a long period of time. Examples of this noxious influence includes geopathic radiation, electrical installations, television sets and heating cables in the floor.

Geopathic radiation can create the same kind of susceptibility in trees. An example of this is the tendency for trees under this stress to be hit by lightning more often than other trees in adjacent areas. Similar to the behavior of electrical currents, lightning-bolts tend to seek the "path of least resistance" through the air. The exact places where they hit the ground are not random; they are places where electrical resistance is the lowest, and likewise where conductivity is highest.

Trees that are struck by lightning usually are directly over, or very close to geopathic lines. These geopathic lines can be created by water flow beneath the earth. Oak trees like to grow near underground water, therefore this species tends to have a greater percentage of lightning strikes. Similarly, Elder trees thrive in damp places, especially on river-banks, and are also under the same kind of geopathic stress.

On Animals.

In my practice, I have found it almost impossible to treat animals or humans successfully if they remain exposed to a precipitating stressor, such as geopathic radiation. In contrast, my clinical results improve greatly if I can show the owner or subject how to avoid these geopathic stressors thereby helping to keep the immune system robust.

Animals free to roam at will seem to avoid areas of noxious radiation. This also appears to be the case for most domestic animals. However, some animals are often forced to stay for prolonged periods in or over areas of adverse electromagnetic fields or geopathic radiation. This can cause geopathic stress which, as with plants, can contribute to illness. Cows exposed chronically to geopathic radiation are less likely to thrive and have shown to be more vulnerable to infection, ketosis and infertility. However, some cows on the point of calving often choose to seek these zones as a place to give birth to their calves.

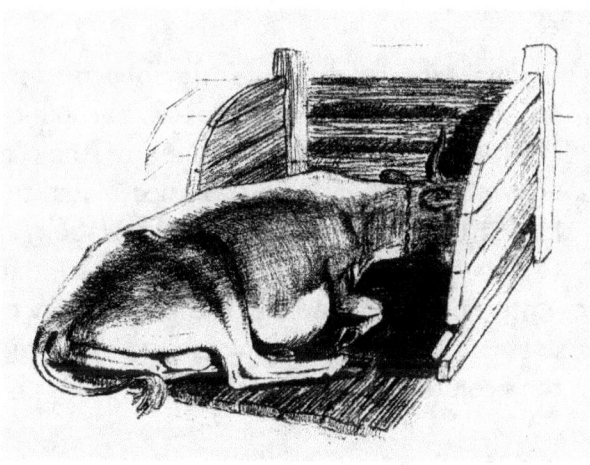

Cow lying over geopathic radiation

Certain animals, such as owls, bats and cats, seek out areas of strong radiation for their dwelling places. Traditionally, according to folklore, these particular animals have been associated with dark powers. Certain insects, such as ants, bees, and wasps also exhibit this same "radiophilic" behavior. For example, it has been shown that swarms of bees often settle in trees that are growing over strong areas of radiation. In addition, beehives placed over crossing aquifers produce more honey than hives placed away from these zones.

Ants often, after exiting the nest, immediately follow paths of geopathic radiation, and travel in the same path as that which can be dowsed. Experiments were done by Rupert Sheldrake, to shield ants' nests from geopathic radiation. The results demonstrated that they left the nest the following year. Therefore, he concluded that ants preferred not to stay for the winter in a nest that was not under the influence of this kind of radiation. A possible explanation theorized that a nest over a strong dowsing zone also was associated with an underground water source.[56]

From personal experience, I have often observed that people bitten by mosquitoes are attacked at the exact acupuncture point that would be appropriate for treatment of their diagnosed imbalance. From this observation, I have postulated that insects relate to this Earth radiation. As this radiation can cause pathology, it can be deduced that insects are attracted to disease. In addition, Anthroposophy states that the pathology created by geopathic stress is under Ahriman's influence, which is the catalyst for the evolution of the 8th sphere[57].

---

[57] **The Occult Movement in the Nineteenth Century, Occult Movement: Lecture Five, GA 254.** The 8th sphere is not a particularly well-known concept, even among those who are students of the study of the Spiritual world. For those familiar with the concept, it can seem quite frightening. Essentially, the 8th sphere is considered the planet where all Ahrimanic deeds, thoughts and concepts materialize in a separate physical world that will, in the far future, be left behind by the common and continued development of the universe and human kind. It is the final depot for those without a consciousness that have created serious misdeeds. It may also be the final depot for those of us who fall prey to a soul-less attraction to the lifeless and artificial. This includes synthetic drugs, additives, pharmaceutical medicines and artificial food. Other lures include our preoccupation within the field of computer technology, a world of soul-less and life-less machines. This also includes those who mindlessly partake in functions requiring the use of computers, such as discussions on Facebook, conversations through e-mails and all lifeless computer interactions where the soul cannot enter nor participate. The consequences are ominous regarding the abuse of technology. Many occultists have spoken and written about the 8th sphere, with many variations and even more oppositional theories regarding what it is, where it is, and how it is organized. Rudolf Steiner had his own opinions and gave several lectures that mentioned the 8th sphere[57]. In these lectures, he emphasizes that it actually belongs to our physical earth. As we create the illusion of the material world, we create a denser material, a density far greater than other mineral substances. This sphere circles around earth as a globe of dense matter, solid and indestructible unable to be dissolved by Lucifer and Ahriman.

Human Involvement in Geopathic Radiation

Even if "normal" animals avoid geopathic radiation, they often follow such lines for their pathways. Recent investigations carried out by dowsers, appear to demonstrate that these geopathic lines are created only where man or animals travel. A simple explanation for this was born of a theory that if plant growth is smaller along these lines, it would be natural for animals to move around where it is easiest to pass. Therefore, the relationship between man's path and the radiation line is because he is simply choosing the path of least resistance. Therefore, one cannot say that they follow the radiation path but, rather, they choose the path of least resistance. However, there is increasingly more evidence and observations indicating that the geopathic radiation is created by the activities of humans themselves.

For example, the dowsers of long ago believed that nearly all of the old churches were built over or were in strict relation to ley-lines or other patterns of geopathic radiation. The same was also found in relation to old trails, roads, burial sites and places of worship. To investigate this, a group of Scandinavian dowsers, including myself, followed closely the development of all energetic patterns relating to newly built churches and roads. We then discovered something amazing; the grid of radiation was organized and created as the construction proceeded. The area where a new church was to be built could be totally clean and free from Earth-Radiation, but after the church was built, the entire radiation pattern, usually seen only in connection with ancient churches, again was present.

Once I experience the same phenomenon at a biodynamic farm in Vestfold, Norway. The farmer, Asbjørn Lavoll, was investigating the effect of different natural fertilizers. I helped him find an area clear of geopathic radiation to eliminate that variable in his experiment. I stood there, watching as Lavoll proceeded with his investigations. But, as soon as he lined up the different squares that were used in the trial, I visualized the appearance of a strong pattern of radiation. I innately realized that this pattern of radiation was related to the planet Saturn and to the metal lead. Such patterns are often created when a materialistic way of thinking excludes a more Spiritual way of thinking. The intention of the farmer to make rectangular squares in which he was to compare the effect of different Spiritually prepared fertilizers, expressed itself as an Ahrimanic grid (demon of material thinking), which draws its force from Saturn. This is a classic example of the observation in quantum physics that no experiment can be completely objective if the outcome is influenced by the mind of the searcher. Using this framework, I argue that the source of these ley lines is the human mind.

As is the case with animals, excessive Earth radiation affects humans adversely. Hundreds of disorders caused by noxious geopathic radiation can be found in the dowsing literature of various countries. These diseases include insomnia, neurasthenia, depression, sudden infant death syndrome, asthma, arthralgia, arthritis, cancer, and other degenerative diseases such as multiple sclerosis. I have seen many examples of this in my practice.

Examples of Pathology caused by Earth radiation

I have treated children who would cry non-stop, until I asked the parents to move their beds, often as little as 0.5 meters. The crying would often cease immediately after the bed was repositioned. I have also treated several patients with chronic ulcers and infections that heal quickly after such a repositioning.

An elderly gentleman came to me after a small splinter in his finger became infected. He was given antibiotics, but the infection continued to the point that the finger was removed. In horror, the patient watched the infection continue to travel up his arm followed by continued dissection of the entire arm. Relentlessly, the infection went further up into the face. In desperation, he appeared at my office with a missing arm, a distorted face, and in terrible distress. I discovered that he was under the strong influence from the geopathic radiation of a local demon, which weakened the etheric and astral fields of his right side. I strengthened the auras and asked him to move away from the place where he was sleeping. Although the disease had gone on for several months, the next morning, the infection was substantially diminished, and after a few weeks, the entire infection resolved. As this local Demon resonated in appearance with the opportunistic contagion, it accelerated the pace and intensity of his condition.

Chronic Exposure to Electrical Magnetic Fields as a Cause of Cancer.

The United States National Cancer Institute stated on May 27, 2016 that many studies and scientific reviews have evaluated possible associations between exposure to non-ionizing EMFs and risk of cancer in children. Most of the research was on leukemia and brain tumors, the two most common cancers in children. Studies have examined associations of these cancers with living near power lines, magnetic fields in the home, and exposure of parents to high levels of magnetic fields in the workplace. However, according to the research findings of the N.C.I., no consistent evidence for an association between any source of non-ionizing EMF and cancer had been found. I view this statement with some skepticism due to a societal bias based on our dependency on electrical power. One could only imagine the mass hysteria awoken by the announcement that everything that emits an electrical current could be leading to our demise. Most governments would be hesitant to sound such an alarm. Without electric power, mass unemployment, social unrest and anarchy would destroy the economic and social cohesion of modern societies.

The Relationship Between Chronic Exposure to Electromagnetic Fields and Brain Tumors.

This is an excerpt from an e-mail that I received from an Irish colleague;

> "Some years ago, death rate from cancer in workers in a large national research institute was noted to be far above that in the general population. The institute had several laboratories in different parts of Ireland. An investigation was conducted to determine if the deaths could be work-related. The team included a medical doctor who specialized in environmental medicine and Trade Union representatives from each of the labs involved. I was one of the investigators. We searched for a possible link of this death rate to exposure to lab reagents, gases, chemicals, carcinogens and nuclear materials. However, we could not find a satisfactory reason to explain the abnormal death rate. In one lab, two genetically unrelated scientists had died within a short interval of each other. The cause of death in both cases was a rare brain tumor. Both men worked in adjoining offices. The fuse-box for the lab's power supply was just outside the wall of one office and multiple power cables from that fuse-box ran directly over the heads of both men. The doctor discounted any causality between the cancer in both men and their concomitant exposure to this electrical field. Although I am an experienced veterinary researcher, not qualified in human medicine, I disagree with the investigator's conclusion. I am convinced that my colleagues died due to cancer triggered by EMFs emitted by the power cables."

Energy Production, Geopathic Radiation and The Elementals.

When humans produce artificial energy from electricity, nuclear energy, wind turbines, and solar energy, benevolent elementals are either changed into demons, or new demons are created. A perfect example of this is the plight of wind elementals. These entities can be trapped by wind turbines, and changed, by the nature of the technology, to demonic ahrimanic elementals. I have seen many examples of how the creation of such destructive elementals from wind-turbines or even worse from solar panels has created almost unrepairable damage relating to both disease, death and social problems in the communities where such energy production has been established. It is important to keep such production furthest away from where man and animals live as possible.

Old sources of energy (those predating the invention of electrical power), such as burning wood, coal and oil, attracts specific elementals called "Salamanders". When using this kind of energy, they remain in a benign elemental form. A demon can only be created when magnetism, electricity or nuclear power is the source of our energy.

According to the ancient texts: fire, air, earth and water are considered the basic elements of nature. Within each of the four Elements, there are three levels of Elemental Beings, categorized as "the first kingdom", "the second kingdom" and the "third kingdom". The beings of the third realm are referred to as *Nature Spirits*. All the Elemental Beings of all three realms are considered the *Spiritual Essence* of that element. The Elementals are made up of an Etheric substance that is unique and specific to their particular element. The Entities of this third realm (the nature spirits) are living entities often resembling humans in shape but inhabiting a world of their own. The Elemental Beings in the elemental kingdoms work primarily on the mental plane and are known as *"Builders of Form"*. Their specialty is to translate Thought-Forms into physical forms by transforming Spiritual patterns into first Astral patterns, then Etheric patterns and then finally physical patterns. Each of them is a specialist in creating some specific form whether it is an electron or interstellar space. Elementals range in size from something smaller than an electron to objects vaster than galactic space. Like the Angels, Elemental Beings begin their evolution small in stature and increase in size as they evolve. The Elementals serving on planet earth materialize whatever they pick up from the thoughts and feelings of mankind. This relationship was intended to facilitate the re-manifestation of "heaven on earth". They do not remain as individualized as humans. They may be etheric thought forms, yet they have etheric flesh, blood, and bones. They live, eat, talk, act and sleep. They cannot be destroyed by material elements such as fire, air, earth and water because they are etheric in nature. They are not immortal. When their work is finished they are absorbed back into the ocean of the Spirit world. They live a rather long time from 300 to 1,000 years and have the power to change their size and appearance at will. They cannot, however, change into other elements.

The Effect of Electricity on the Elementals

As stated earlier, Elementals are the Spiritual foundation of nature and are also created by human deeds. When electricity was created, this process created a host of demonic Elementals, entities detrimental to the harmony of the existing benign spirits and their relationship with humans.

In 2015, I visited an Amish community in New York State. One of the peculiarities about the Amish people is that they do not use electricity. Before I visited them, I thought that the Elementals always were a rather ambivalent lot with no interest in humans.

This opinion changed after seeing the behavior of an elemental in an Amish community. Here, I was greeted by smiling and engaging forms of this faction. I was both touched and shaken by this observation, now understanding the terrible effect that electricity has on these Spirit beings.

In contrast, I read an article from an interview with a Native American Indian explaining the opposite situation in which he said, *"after we got electricity here in the camp, we do not hear the Spirits of Nature speaking to us any more …."*.

Another example of this phenomenon revolves around a village in middle Norway whose inhabitants had certain problems with their social life and health. I was asked to visit to see if I could find the cause of these problems. As I was approaching the village, I started to observe a strange change in all the houses I passed. They appeared to be divided in two parts, one smaller darkened part and one larger vibrant part. What was even more peculiar was that all the houses were divided in the same way, even houses that were unoccupied. This peculiarity continued all the way to the village, and in the center, it was even more predominant. I was then sure that this was the origin of the problems. When exiting the car, I stood for a moment and looked around. And then I spotted it; a huge windmill, placed in the middle of the village. As this windmill was supplying all the village's energy, the leaders were quite proud of their environmentally sound investment. However, in reality, the windmill was also creating hordes of malevolent elementals of the demonic kind. These creations were what was causing the strange division of all the village structures.

Electro-Magnetic Radiation, can the harm be neutralized – or can it even be made beneficial?

For many years and through many investigations, it has been shown that electro-magnetic radiation (EMR) can harm living beings such as plants, animals and humans. When we look at this harm, we find that it is, especially relating to humans, quite individual.

Over the past decade, we find that more and more human beings react to EMR with allergic symptoms; again, this is fully individual.

Rudolf Steiner has in countless lectures, books, and conversations underlined that the two great adversaries of our time, Lucifer and Ahriman, are actually placed here by God to help us in our development. In fact, in the future, they will serve as part of a new trinity.

Steiner speaks of electricity as light-ether that has been pressed into the sub-earthly realms where it is as if frozen until it can later emerge as what we know as electricity.

This energy-form is used as a vehicle by Lucifer.

Magnetism is today an effect of the chemical ether being pressed into the sub-earthly realms, frozen and then emerges as what we know as magnetism. This energy-form is used as a vehicle by Ahriman. Together, through their demonic forces or their demons they are able to hurt life, create disease and cause cancer.

We are not supposed to fight these forces.

If we do so we just push or even strengthen the demonic forces or demons, and nothing will be attained. Even diseases treated in all our different ways will just be translocated to other living beings if not treated or dealt with in a transformative way.

Many people who work in the field of isolating houses against malevolent earth radiation, have to change the devices frequently, often once a month.

We have the choice between translocation and transformation of the described forces. We can flee from them by changing the place of the bed, translocate them through various devices such as copper, keep away from them, or really transform them through an understanding of what these forces are and where they come from.

The pathological and malevolent effects from electromagnetic radiation are caused by the adversarial forces "riding" the electromagnetic wave from which they can be separated. Then the pathological effect of the electromagnetic radiation disappear, hypersensitivity will vanish, and we can use electricity or EMR in a healthy way.

As far as I have found, two other persons have worked with the idea of splitting off the pathological adversarial forces from the EMR, and thus render it harmless.

- **Ibrahim Karim**. He uses his techniques to separate what he terms toxic vertical waves from EM radiation leaving the non-toxic and perhaps beneficial horizontal waves. https://fmbr.org/science-of-biogeometry/
- **Emanuel Blosser** of Edmonton, Alberta, several years ago noted from his own spiritual research that individuals who performed significant effort to spiritual activity could ward off the negative effects of EMR. Knowledge frees the counter forces from bondage to mineral matter.

An explanation from homeopathy

In homeopathy we can see and understand that the spiritual powers or demonic force can be separated from the physical material or physical radiation.

Homeopaths describe what is left in the remedy as the "information structure of the substance", a kind of "resonance" or hidden information.

Homeopaths suggest that succussion induces a structural change in the water molecules where there exists a surface tension layer between water and bubbles. In this way, the remedy-free vehicle preserves the information structure or therapeutic signal of the remedy that induces its clinical effect. According to Avogadro's law, the number of molecules in 1 g of any homeopathic substance is less than 6×10^{23}. When we dilute any substance 24 times at 1:10 each time (i.e. D24), the concentration becomes 1×10^{-24}.

Theoretically there are no molecules left in the solution at that dilution. In practice, it is not possible to detect the substance at higher dilutions such as D7 orD8. Conventional medicine classifies homeopathic remedies above D6 as having no possible toxic effect. At least it cannot reject homeopathic remedies on grounds of toxicity or lack of safety.

From my experiences with spirits, adversarial elementals, demonic structures of luciferic and ahrimanic origin and "set-free-demons", I know that succussion [you will need to define this term] also has another effect on the spiritual content of any substance.

The characteristics of the elemental beings within the medical plant used for making the remedy looks very much like the pathological being that causes the disease. This is the basis of the homeopathic law of "similia similibus curentur". Homeopaths know or postulate that the energy of the plant or the metal mysteriously translocates into the water when the dilution is shaken. This shaking enables the spirit of the healing plant to enter or translocate into the remedy. This is then called potentiation; it makes the water "potent".

For example, the spiritual effect or activity in arsenic, arsenicum, can, in homeopathy, be divided from the physical substance of arsenicum, and thus be used as a medicine, while the toxic substance can be thrown away.

Of course this translocated spirit of the medical plant, often called the demon of the plant as the medical plant often is toxic and the plant-spirit then often looks very "demonic" [looks to whom? Clairvoyant sight], can further translocate the demon of the disease itself. This is described by Dr. Constantin Hering which of course is the law of translocation.

The middle-point of cosmos, solar system, earth, humans and all material things

The Middle-point is a new concept of treatment and the solution to changing the EMR into first something unharmful and then into something good.

In 2016, I understood clearly that I could not use acupuncture according to the normal Chinese thinking to treat cancer as the cancer then just translocated to another human being or an animal. I then decided to try employing the Middle Point. I discovered this point by studying the works of **Judith von Halle**. She states that a diseased patient should be healed using "Christ-Consciousness". I was still in confusion: how do I treat with "Christ consciousness"? After looking carefully at the wooden sculpture called "The Group" or "The Representative of Man", made by **Rudolf Steiner** and **Edith Maryon**, depicting Christ standing between the two dominating adversarial and pathological entities, Lucifer and Ahriman, I realized that the healthy energy of the Christ consciousness lies between these; yin and yang structures residing in the body. I named the loci that could accomplish this task the "Middle Point".

Using this point, I treat neither the excess nor the deficiency, but try to stimulate the middle or healthy area that lies between these two opposites. Since 2014, I have treated many human and veterinary patients with the Middle Point; that is, as single patients using one needle carefully placed in the middle, or with my fingers held in the gesture that Christ has in the group-statue made by Edith Maryon and Rudolf Steiner, pushing the luciferic and the ahrimanic entities apart, making way for the Christ force to enter. Most patients seem to be satisfied with the effect of this treatment.

- The yang structures are always proximal or cranial, in the front and to the right.

- The yin structures are almost always distal (in animals caudal), at the back and to the left.
- The Christ consciousness lies between them. In my book, *Spiritual Medicine*, this is discussed in detail.

This middle Christ-force is three-fold, it exists in three dimensions.

- The luciferic forces are more to the head, to the right and to the front.
- The ahrimanic forces are more to be found towards the pelvis, to the left and to the back.

In this way we must widen and strengthen the Christ-force in all directions, as a sphere that is enlarged, just as depicted by Michelangelo in his picture shown above "Salvatore Mundi".

This middle can be treated in many ways, whereof I find the best to be the manual method. I hold my hands in the area of the middle, imagining it to be like the sphere Christ is holding in the picture painted by Michelangelo, and then enlarge is between my hands.

Since I discovered the middle-point in living humans and animals, I have for several years tried to find the Middle Point also in "dead" man-made devices. Contrary to belief that these devices are "dead", they are creations of the human mind, and are thus endowed with a form of elemental life. They also contain the elemental forces of the luciferic- and the ahrimanic realm, without which the material existence would not be possible. They also have the midpoint, the Christ-point between the two forces.

Description of how a separation of the adversarial forces from the EMR

Two examples:

- With this knowledge of EMR, I did the following experiment. In Germany, at a horse center there were 14 horses, all of which were lame to different degrees. However, all of them had pain in the spleen area be-tween the 16th and the 18th rib at the back, and this pain had then caused the different types of lameness. Just 100 meters from the stable there was a G4 mast. The EMR radiation from this mast could be felt very strongly, and it was obvious that this EMR made the horses sick. I had gathered a group of 12 people, and at a distance of approximately 50 meters we all attempted to mentally push apart the forces of the adversaries abiding in the mast, and thereby create a space for the Middle Point, the Christ-force. After 10 minutes all pain in the back of the horses was gone and within a few days all of them were free of lameness. I checked the situation 2 years later and everything was still fine in this stable. The pathological aspect of the radiation was gone, although the mobile phones still worked. The spiritual was separated from the material. This treatment was done by people that did not "see" the spiritual elementary beings.
- Some colleagues and I sat in a restaurant that was "rigged up" with about 20 television sets, each showing their separate program. All who were eating sat like zombies and just put the food in their mouths whilst their eyes were focused deep into the television emissions. I related the incidence of the horse experience in Germany to my colleagues, and then I proceeded to make the following experiment: Concentrating on one of the TVs I separated the ahrimanic and luciferic powers, and almost immediately there was a significant change in the people who were watching this particular one. Suddenly they became humanized, taking an interest in the food they

were putting in their mouths, becoming alive in their movements, talking together and showing obvious changes in their behavior.

This subject is of utmost importance both now and in the years to come. Today we all are under a very severe attack from electromagnetic radiation. This radiation comes from 4G-masts, 5G-masts, Cell-phones and all kinds of electro-magnetic devices.

I have tried, with 4G-masts, with TV-sets and with cell-phones to concentrate my willing and intending mind on the middle-point of these devices, expand this middle-point and thus weaken the adversarial forces. Using this kind of 'treatment", I have observed a marked effect on the allergic pathologies of the people and animals affected by EMR.

Sensitivity coming from EM-devices, the "allergic" reactions to radiation and the resulting physical pain have completely disappeared after such a concentrated effort, after such a 'treatment" of only 10 minutes. How can this be possible?

If we think about the making of homeopathic remedies, we 'split" to a certain extent the physical remedy from the 'spiritual" remedy, and use the spiritual part as the medical remedy, without having to care about the toxic effects of the material substance.

It is then also possible to 'split" the toxic part of the radiation from the devices described, the part that belongs to the adversaries, to Lucifer and Ahriman, and just keep the "functional" part, which is the TV-pictures, the Cell-phone-conversation or the electric heating of a house.

In such a partial splitting we have to use our willing mind, where the divided willing is first led down into the earth and then allowed to rise up again. At the halfway point it must be met by the intending thoughts of the mind, and in this meeting of will and intent, a force is created to split the pathological from the physical, at least to such a degree that the pathological effect of the radiation disappears.

To repeat: I consider the middle to be the only force of reality, our only salvation. Our "logical" conception of reality in making everything into polarities, is for me like being dragged into Maya, the Maya of illusion.

The polarities seem to me to be an expression of this great illusion, whilst the trinity expresses the reality. It is of vital importance to find this third aspect in all uses of electricity, magnetism, nuclear power, cosmic streams or corporeal balances, otherwise the ahrimanic-luciferic forces will dominate.

We find the same opposition between duality and trinity in the soul forces of thinking, feeling and willing. Within each we must find the Middle Point, the middle force of love. If we can then relate to and use this middle force, this power of LOVE as a fourth stream permeating the cosmos, we will be victorious. We have a cosmic cross, expressed by the morning-evening-midday-midnight forces. Our only salvation is to add the force of LOVE to the fundamental forces of thinking, feeling and willing. That is why the cross is a symbol reflecting the love of Jesus Christ.

The beneficial effect of the "free" EMR

As **Ibrahim Karin** suggest in his work, the "free" EMR can, contrary to many beliefs, work beneficial or healing in relation to disease and human well-being.

I have now, after having "split" the adversarial forces from the EMR for several years, stated to see beneficial health effects from this radiation, almost in the same way that the "free" spirituality of homeopathic remedies can heal diseases.

This is an area that must be further investigated.

The Relationship of Specific Energy Sources to Specific Demons and Their Related Diseases

Rudolf Steiner has described the connection of varying energy sources in relation to the elemental and demonic realms: He has lectured that electricity creates and fuels ahrimanic demons. Luciferic demons are formed and fueled by magnetism, while nuclear power awakens and nourishes those of the Azuric nature. All three of these energy sources lead to strengthening of their respective doppelgänger or demon.

In this connection, it is interesting to note how electricity and magnetism is used in the healing of different diseases in humans and animals. Magnets and Electrical therapeutic devices sometimes work wonders, especially in cases of rheumatic pain and related musculoskeletal ailments. However, more often than not, they prove to be worthless toward a long term sustainable cure.

The reason for this this is due to the adversarial relationship between ahrimanic and luciferic demons in the creation and development of disease. Magnetic devices can cure symptoms caused by ahrimanic demons, because luciferic demons counteract the effects of the ahrimanic doppelgänger. Similarly, electric devices can cure symptoms caused by luciferic demons because ahrimanic demons counteract the effects of luciferic demons.

This may also be why marijuana is reported to "work" beneficially in some diseases but fails to help in others. It even works differently on the same symptoms in different people. This is because marijuana strengthens the luciferic demons and this may counteract the ahrimanic symptoms. However, only Christ's consciousness can treat both, thus evoking a truly curative response, and a direct influence on the doppelgängers or the demons will likely lead to translocation.

The use of Technology and its Role in Demonology: The role of the 12 sense organs

In anthroposophy, the sense organs play an important role as a connection between the physical and spiritual words. In the physical world, we are all aware of our five sense organs, However, according to Rudolf Steiner there are actually 12.

This is due to the fact that we must now include the entire makeup of man as seen through the "spiritual eye". Our sensory organs are not only from openings from the physical body, but also include ethereal and astral portals between our inner world and the cosmos.

I would conjecture that most people believe that the explosion of technological advances has been the heralding of an era of a profound evolution. With the push of a few buttons, anything and everything can be found, researched, bought and sold. In addition, our ability to immediately connect with one another through social media has morphed the concept of the written word. Language has now taken on a divisiveness of monumental proportions, as the "insta-word" has assumed the role of becoming the most effective weapon since the invention of the gun. So, it is no wonder that the existence of electronic technology has also created an effective tool for the blossoming of adversarial forces. This book will explain the exact methodology in which Ahriman, as the primary sinister force, can manipulate the devices of this technology to gain control over the future of humanity. His major access point is through the portals created by our sense organs

Rudolf Steiner has thoroughly described the existence of 12 senses[58]. He claimed that each of these faculties act as openings or portals to both the physical, etheric and astral aspects of both man

---

[58] Steiner, Rudolf; The Twelve Human Senses, Berlin, June 20, 1916

and the cosmos in which we live. Each sense is connected to one of the divine beings of the first hierarchy, expressed in each of the 12 signs of the zodiac. In this way, they can be viewed as a 12-fold entity

In Steiner's description of human beings, he categorizes our make-up using several methods. First, he divides us into 4 layers, consisting of our physical, etheric, astral and "I" sheaths. However, this concept of a four-fold being can be further described as having both 7 and even 9 levels, if one also considers our spiritual future as including the higher levels named Budi, Manas, and Atma. Ultimately, our higher selves, as well as all of creation, are governed by a primary trinity of the powerful soul faculties of Thinking, Feeling and Willing. They represent the fundamental processes in which our cosmos is organized and developed and weave themselves into all aspects of creation. This trinity encompasses the entire cosmos, the divine angelic hierarchies, as well as the "under-nature" world of spiritual beings such as elves, hidden people and other elementals. This latter aspect of our universe can be seen with the spiritual eye as an upside-down reality of the physical world (or perhaps it could be our world that is upside down). In this way, one can imagine as if our feet were to make contact with their reverse image beneath the spiritual earth.

The three cosmic forces play a role in every aspect of our lives. They are revealed within the anthroposophical medical system as the three fundamental poles of the nerve-sensory system (thinking), the rhythmic system (feeling) and the metabolic/ muscular/ skeletal system (willing)[59]. However, it is of paramount importance, that we understand that this template also can be applied to the 12 senses, particularly when we are considering the steps toward spiritual initiation known as imagination (the 4

---

[59] Rudolf Steiner and Ita Wegman, Extending Practical Medicine: Rudolf Steiner Press, 2000

physical senses of touch, life, movement and orientation), inspiration (the 4 soul-senses of smell, taste, temperature and sight), and intuition (the 4 spiritual senses of hearing, speech, thought and perception of the "I" of others).

The senses described by Steiner are extremely complex formations as they exhibit both an outward and inward direction of flow. For example, the eyes which perceive the cosmos, are sending an outward etheric stream enabling them to also receive an inward flow of information from what they are viewing. It is a general spiritual rule that any movement automatically creates a counter movement, even involving time.

The 12 senses are also developed in the Luciferic, Ahrimanic, and human karmic Doppelgängers. These three entities employ the senses in a unique way. The human karmic doppelgänger uses the physical sense organs as we use them in the material world. The Ahrimanic and Luciferic doppelgängers, however, create their own mirror images of these structures. The template that Ahrimanic forces utilize are situated deeper within the physical body, while the Luciferic templates are more superficial, infiltrating the Astral sheath. For example, in the eye, the Ahrimanic sense organ lies about 1cm behind the material optic structure while the Luciferic is in front of the eye. I perceive the Ahrimanic structure with my clairvoyant ability as a grayish structure, similar to a tin plate.

These structures are also activated and developed by viewing electronic screens. From this information, it can be surmised that there are actually three aspects of each of these sense organs. If one considers all 12 sense organs and combines the fact that all these senses are employed by three doppelgängers (including ourselves), and that each organ is involved in both an outgoing and an ingoing stream, we come to the conclusion that we are actually dealing with 72 qualities that must be considered when understanding sensory function. Note that all 12 senses can create a spiritual observation. For example, if the spiritual eye is developed, we refer to that ability as clairvoyance.

The first sense I will discuss is the eye, the foundation of sight and also very central in imagination and clairvoyance. Regarding the eye as a physical organ, I have observed that when viewing a living object, especially in nature, the inhabitants of higher spiritual hierarchies are also sharing the observation. I have also found that the sense organs with little or no fat, such as the eye, have a stronger affinity for the etheric. However, when one is observing the screen of a cell phone, the observations are intertwined with another reality where colors diminish and Ahrimanic forces dominate.

Regarding the effect of the presence of the effects of Lucifer and Ahriman on our sense organ of sight, whether we are observing the results of these demonic influences on the nature of the physical world, or on the under-nature of the virtual electronic world, I find that both demons can thrive on the latter, including the internet, artificial light, LED displays, computer monitors and cell phones. This is described in the books of Paul Emberson, "From Gondshapur to Silicon Valley". While the adversaries such as Lucifer and Ahriman will be able to take part in this under-world via electronics, handwriting is a safer alternative for communication as it is under the domain of the Angels.

The strength of these doppelgängers is weaved into the sensory observations. Paul Emberson claims that the use of computers stimulates the adversarial forces strong hold on our existence. For example, if one views a movie, he will actually strengthen the Ahrimanic doppelgänger's visual sense organ. As mentioned above, this eye is grey and large, similar in appearance to a plate made of tin. In 1917, Steiner addresses his concern about attending a movie theater.[60] He describes that the eyes of those

---

[60] Cosmic and Human Metamorphoses, Steiner, Rudolf; lecture 4, 1917: " while people are sitting at the cinema, what they see there does not make its way into the ordinary faculty of perception, it enters a deeper, more material stratum than we usually employ for our perception. A man becomes etherically goggle-eyed at the cinema; he develops eyes like those of a seal, only much larger, I mean larger etherically. This works in a materialising way, not only upon what he has in his consciousness, but upon its deepest sub-consciousness".

watching a movie film take on the sense organs of Ahriman. An interesting inference to such an eye in literature can be found in the famous Henrik play entitled "Peer Gynt". A surgery is described where a slit is made in the eye to "fake" the adversarial forces into thinking that everything the person saw was beautiful to assure a marriage of the Troll king's daughter.

The second sense I would like to discuss is that of feeling. The related organ to this sense at the physical level is the skin. My observations regarding this organ dates back to well before my understanding of anthroposophy. During the first years of my veterinary studies at Oslo University, I spent some time between classes observing the tourists, especially those that were overweight. I saw, with my spiritual eye that, in many of those people, the skin was in front of a withdrawn etheric sheath. The fatty tissue was in a way hanging loose, out of the etheric field. In this way, the effect of the sense organ allowing *clairsentience,* was diminished. In other words, weight can have an effect on supra-sensory feeling. Therefore, when a person goes on a weight reduction program, they may be possible to develop their spiritual sense of touch as the etheric sheath expands in an outward direction, thus diminishing the stranglehold of Ahriman and Lucifer on this particular sense organ. This might be why Christ fasted as he resisted the temptations of these demons during his 40 days in the desert. Being thinner perhaps allowed him to attain a higher level of spirituality.

When the physical sense organ of the skin is involved, as well as its Luciferic and Ahrimanic templates, we must understand how Rudolf Steiner described clairvoyance as a relationship between the physical body, etheric body and astral body, especially when the spiritual bodies are outside the physical form. For example, during the time of Atlantis, the etheric sheath of the head was outside its physical counterpart. In this way Atlanteans were clairvoyant and able to observe the etheric world. However, if the etheric body is within the physical body, the super sensible sense organs become muted

Therefore, it appears that the Ahrimanic and Luciferic sense organs are developing in synch with our growing love of technology, especially over the past 20 years. As Goethe wrote that the sun created the need for our human eyes, so will the existence of virtual media and electronic devices create the need for an Ahrimanic eye.

I have observed that children are developing a special affinity for understanding and partaking in such devices, as the doppelgänger eye becomes more sophisticated. The healthy spiritual forces, in contrast, avoid such devices creating a dissolution of healthy social connections among the populous. An even more sinister connotation lies in the inability for us to advance our goal toward spiritual initiation through the process of imagination, inspiration, and intuition. Therefore, we must proceed with caution to limit electronic communications in our daily life by restraining from using e mail, face book and other such forms of social media. Our soul life, etheric life, and our physical bodies depend on it. We must protect our future now, whether it be for our children but also for the future of the spirit of humanity as a whole.

Earlier in this book, we learned that there are three soul faculties of Thinking, Feeling and Willing that, when separated, relate to the development of Imagination, Inspiration and Intuition. Imagination relates to the sensory organs of the transformed physical body, Inspiration to the soul sensory organs, and Intuition to the spiritual sensory organs.

Listed below are these unique organ categories

- Four sensory organs associated with the physical
    - touch, expressed in the skin.
    - life, expressed in the mucous membranes.
    - movement, expressed in the muscles.
    - orientation, is expressed in the inner ear

- Four sensory organs associated with the soul
    - smell, expressed in the nose.
    - taste, expressed in the tongue.
    - temperature expressed in the skin.
    - visual sensibilities, expressed in the eyes.

- Four sensory organs associated with the spirit:
    - hearing, expressed in the inner ear.
    - word comprehension, expressed in the movement system.
    - thoughts, expressed in the life-sense.
    - feeling for 'others', expressed in the etheric skin.

The detail explanation of these 12 sense organs is beyond the scope of this text and can be further investigated by studying the works of Anthroposophy. However, the reader should keep in mind the importance of the portals these special organs in receiving both beneficial and harmful information from the Spirit World.

Paul Emberson, a noted anthroposophist, stated in his book, *"From Gondishapur to Silicon Valley"*, that any information transmitted by electricity, magnetism, or quantum physics, will be tainted by adversarial forces, whereas writing by hand will allow the entry of the higher hierarchies. In the same vein, I have noticed that when a person observes nature, the higher spiritual forces join in the observation. However, when the person looks at his smartphone, the color-sensing processes in the eye move to another dimension. The natural colors disappear and our Ahrimanic Double weaves itself into our sensory observation.

Paul Emberson also claims that by using computers, powerful adversarial forces can weave into our lives. For example, if we are watching a movie, our eyes will change into "Ahrimanic" eyes, similar to "tin plates" as described in some mythical accounts of aliens.

Thus, new Ahrimanic "copies" of our sense organs are developing in line with humanity's use of them. These Ahrimanic sensory organs seem to be more developed today than 20 years ago. I believe the existence of the electromagnetic and virtual media will help to evolve these aberrant organ forms. Children are now seemingly born with an innate recognition and understanding of the virtual worlds. Sadly, the good forces will no longer participate in the impressions conveyed through these new sensory organs, and we will lose the impact of these beneficial forces in our healthy conversations. In addition, since initiation through Imagination, Inspiration and Intuition is associated our sense organs, the adversarial forces will obtain easy access to these spheres, which ultimately can harm all of humanity.

Thus, when we communicate via any form of electronic media, the opposing powers will have access to all aspects of our life, as well as our Initiation path through Imagination, Inspiration and Intuition.

The Double (Doppelgänger), Ahriman and Disease

Rudolf Steiner lectures in St. Gallen about the connection of "The Double", ahrimanic entities, and disease.

> *"And here something is disclosed, that in the future must be followed up if the human race is not to experience endless hindrances and endless horrors. This double about which I have spoken is nothing more or less than the creator of all physical illnesses that emerge spontaneously from within; and to know him fully is the basis of holistic medicine. He is the creator of all illnesses that emerge spontaneously from within, and a brother of his, who is Luciferic, is the creator of all neurasthenic, neurotic and hysterical illnesses. Thus, medicine must become Spiritual in two directions. The demand for this*

is shown by the intrusion of views such as those of psychoanalysis and the like, where one keeps house with Spiritual entities, as it were, but with inadequate means of knowledge so that one can do nothing at all with the phenomena that will intrude more and more into human life. For certain things need to happen, things that may even be harmful in a certain direction, because the human being must be exposed to what is harmful in order to overcome it and thereby gain strength.

As I have said, this "Ahrimanic Double" is really the creator of all illnesses that have an organ-based foundation that are not merely functional. In order to understand this fully, however, one must know a great deal more. One must know, for example, that our entire earth is not the dead product that mineralogy or geology thinks it to be, but it is a living being. Geology knows as much of the earth as we would know about the human being if we knew only of the skeletal system. Imagine that you were unable to perceive other people with usual sense perception and instead there were only X-rays of our fellow human beings. Then you would know only the skeletal system of your acquaintances. You would know as much about the human being as the geologists and science in general know about the earth. Imagine coming to this lecture and seeing all of the respected ladies and gentlemen you find here as nothing more than bones. Then you would have as much consciousness of the people present here as science has of the earth.

This epoch began in the 15th century, our present period beginning in 1413. The fourth post-Atlantean period, the Greco-Latin, began in 747 B.C. and lasted until 1413. This was a time when a milder incision in history took place. The fifth post-Atlantean epoch began at that *time, and we continue to live in it now. Only gradually is it bringing forth its special characteristics in our time, although these have been in preparation since the fifteenth century. In the 4th post-Atlantean epoch it was chiefly the Intellectual Soul (Verstandes- und Gemütseele) that was developed; now it is the Consciousness Soul that is being developed in the general evolution of humanity. When the human being entered into this epoch, the guiding Spiritual Beings had to consider his special weakness in relation to "The Double". Had the human being taken into his consciousness the knowledge of "The Double", it would have gone badly.*

Before the 14th century, the human being had to be protected, so that he would take in very little of what was suggestive in any way of "The Double". Therefore, the knowledge of this double that existed throughout earlier ages was lost. Humanity had to be guarded so that it would not take up anything of the theory of this double; not only this, however, but it had to come in contact with as little as possible of anything connected with this Double".

The Double and Geography

Rudolf Steiner described the relation of "The Double" (and all ahrimanic beings) to geography (GA 178, St. Gallen, November 15, 1917).

"For this purpose, a very special arrangement was required. You must try to understand what developed at that time. In the centuries preceding the 14th century, the human being had to be guarded from "The Double". The double had to be gradually withdrawn from man's circle of vision. Only now is man gradually permitted to come

into it again, now when the human being must adapt his relationship to "The Double". A really significant arrangement was required, which could be attained only in the following way. Since the 9th or 10th century, conditions in Europe were gradually adjusted in such a way that they lost the connection to America, a connection that was still important for human beings in earlier centuries, the sixth and seventh centuries A.D. Beginning in the 9th century and especially from the 12th century, the entire shipping exchange with America was abolished. This may sound very strange to you. You will say, "We have never heard anything like this in history". In many respects, history is just a fable convenue a legend; for in earlier centuries ships continually sailed from Norway to America. Of course, it was not called America, it had a different name at that time. America was known to be the region where the magnetic forces particularly arose that brought the human being into relation with "The Double". For the clearest relations to "The Double" proceed from that region of the earth that comprises the American continent. In earlier centuries people sailed to America in Norwegian ships and studied illnesses there. The illnesses in America brought about under the influence of earthly magnetism were studied. And the mysterious origin of the older European shamanic medicine is to be sought there. In America, one could observe the course of illness that could not have been observed in Europe, where people were more sensitive with regard to the influence of "The Double". It then became necessary for the connection with America to be gradually forgotten, and this was essentially brought about through the edicts of the Roman Catholic Church.

Only after the beginning of the 5th post-Atlantean epoch was America rediscovered. This was only a rediscovery, however, which is so significant because the powers that were at work actually achieved their purpose: that little would be reported in the record of the ancient relations between Europe and America. Europe had to be protected from the influence of the Western world. This is the significant historical arrangement that was cultivated by wisdom-filled world powers. Europe had to be protected for a long time from all these influences; and it could not have been protected if the European world had not been completely shut off from America in the times before the fifteenth century.

Medicine can endure only if it is a Spiritual science, for illnesses come from a Spiritual Being that only makes use of the human body in order to profit from it, which it cannot do in the place assigned to it by the wise guidance of the world, against which it has revolted, as I have shown you. This is actually an Ahrimanic-Mephistophelian being within the human nature, which before birth is inhaled into the human body and leaves this human body only because it cannot endure death under its present conditions. Illnesses emerge because this being works in the human being. And when remedies are employed it means that something is given to this being from the outer world that it otherwise seeks through the human being. If I provide a remedy for the human body when this Ahrimanic-Mephistophelean being is at work, I give it something else. I stroke this being as it were. I come to terms with it, so that it lets go of the human being and becomes satisfied with what I have tossed into its jaws as a remedy".

Chapter 11:

Quantum-Physics and Spiritual Science

The laws of Quantum Physics and Spiritual Science

The birth of quantum physics forced scientists to rethink their straightforward concepts of reality. Much of the reason for this has to do with the fact that it constructs defies much of the logical thinking of the human mind. The problem is, we are dealing with a subatomic reality, the reality of the immaterial, which is also the reality of the spiritual world. We are no longer viewing the laws of objects but rather of elemental particles. These laws are entirely different; however, quantum physicians integrate the same laws as the spiritual world. Quantum physics challenges us to not only see that things are not what they seem to be, but that they can be anything.

Today, the connection between Christ, Demons (Lucifer, Azuras and Ahriman), the 8th sphere and Quantum-Physics, is of utmost importance.

I believe that Albert Einstein had a deep feeling or intuition about this connection when he said, *"God does not play with dice"*. I get the feeling that Dr. Einstein felt that Quantum-Physics brought in something that is oppositional to God.

The questions that gave birth to theoretical quantum physics came from the idea of spontaneous generation, in other words how does one get something from nothing? From where do these quantum particles emerge?

Paul Emberson, who I mentioned earlier regarding technology and demonology spoke on this question. His conclusions are that our work with and the use of elemental particles and Quantum-Physics, may be a direct opening between our world, the Demonic Azuric world and the 8th sphere.

How can we prove that Quantum-Physics is an opening to the Spiritual world and, in particular, an opening into the Spiritual world of the adversaries? If we were to take a closer look at the fundamental laws of Quantum Physics, we may find that the connection to spiritual science is obvious.

The first law is that of **Entanglement**. This states that particles of the same origin are forever interconnected. Similar to Karma, this is a law of the Spiritual world.

A second law relating to *entanglement* can also be compared to the spiritual world. This law views **time** as a meaningless linear measurement. In quantum physics entanglement between particles is immediate.

The third law, **Non-locality**, relates to the position of the particle in space. The particle can be anywhere and nowhere and it is position can be irrelevant to the reality of the observer. This is particularly important in the classical scientific model of the hypothesis. Because of the variable dynamics of an elementary particle, no two outcomes will be the same.

These three laws described above demonstrate that in Quantum Physics we are dealing with a domain somewhere between the physical and spiritual world. The world I was in during my earlier treatments of cancer when I was able to start seeing the particles of the spirit world that we call demons. It seemed as if every law of quantum physics came into play. I have also come to realize that the spontaneous generation of material particles from seemingly nothing is, more often than not, adversarial beings from the spirit world.

Considering these theories, I have wondered that if the laws of the Spiritual world were truly accepted that there might have been a resolution to the controversies between Niels Bohr and Albert Einstein.

If we use LED-lights and other quantum based physical inventions, we are opening up a path to a future of an Asuric world. This will be in a similar way that we have currently made ourselves susceptible to Ahriman when we employ electricity or Lucifer when we engage in magnetism.

A comparison of the key features of quantum physics to Spiritual Science

The following six principles within physics can explain much about the behavior of Elementals and Demons.

The six principles are:

1. The speed of light (constant in all directions).
2. The equivalence principle (within gravity).
3. The cosmological principle (cosmos is the same in all directions).
4. Quantization (all things are divided in small quantities or packages).
5. Uncertainty (before we see an elemental we don't know how or where it is).
6. Wave-particle duality (all things are both particle or wave).

The first principle is termed "Quantization". This theorem states all things are comprised of a conglomerate of minimal packages. In the spirit world, these are elementals of the first level. The second concept is the "Uncertainty principle". This speaks to the illusion that what we see is predictable. In fact, it is quite the opposite in that the better you "see" the elemental particle (being), the less you can predict where it goes. To take this a step even farther, the more you see the elemental the more it can and will avoid you. This is exactly what I experienced in my cancer therapy, when after long periods of success, "the cancer" seemed to avoid my treatment. That especially occurred when I started to "see" the cancer elementals. To further substantiate this principle, it appeared that as I became more skilled in my ability to see these elementals, the more effective they were in avoiding my treatment. One of the most confounding principles to understand is that of the bipolar nature of the existence of an elemental as both a wave and a particle

Entanglement, a fourth principle, can also be explained using the spiritual concept of an elemental. The elementals are together in the spiritual world and as such, are forever connected. In addition, in their world, time and distance are non-existent. This fourth principle revolves around the speed of light, when such restrictions fade away.

Chapter 12:
The Deep Layers of the Earth and Karma

The Buddhist View of Earth Radiation

The Buddhist view is similar to my experience with the law of karma and radiation. This description is found in the writings of *Sri Ananda Acharia*, a Buddhist monk that immigrated to Norway from India in 1910, and lived his whole life in Alvdal, where he tried to build a university based on peace, love and Buddhism.
In his book *"How Karlima Rani spoke"*, he describes the geopathic radiation as follows; "There are strong forces coming from the cosmos to the earth. These "radiation-energies" change every 2 hours. They may be used in a positive way by living organisms and humans when they are absorbed directly. The radiation from the cosmos is of three types called "Seo', Boom and Beor". If this radiation is not taken into the physical body and used directly, it enters the earth and is then reflected by the Demonic inhabitants of the deeper layers of the earth. It then becomes materialized and changed by the karmic deeds of human beings, and consequently becomes malevolent. This is the origin of Earth-Radiation. It then creates disease".

Earth Radiation of the deeper layers According to Rudolf Steiner

The earth is comprised of the following nine spiritual layers in the same way as man is in his spiritual makeup. Therefore, the earth has its physical form as the crust and the compressed fluid layer. The next layers are etheric and then astral both abundant in astral and etheric life. The eighth layer is a source of evil and from this layer to the ninth the evil increases.

1. The first layer consists of the mineral layer comprised of the outer crust that is employed for the products used the material world.
2. The fluid layer follows this. It is under the constant strain of pressure that exerts an expansive quality toward the surface to be release upward into the cosmos.
3. The third layer is Damp. This is even more expansive than the second layer and is teaming with life. Etherically, it is closely connected with both human passion and the animal world. This includes animalistic emotions such as hunger, greed, violence, killing and despair.
4. The fourth or water layer is Astral in its form. The Astral form is a negative image of the material world (as in a photograph).
5. The fifth earth layer is the seat of pure life. Everything within this layer is alive. The 5th through the 8th layers of the human body mirror the 3de through the 5th of the earth in that both these regions contain an abundant amount of wither astral or etheric life.
6. To continue we come to the sixth layer called the Fire Earth. This layer is also in direct contact with emotions, especially those that tend to be "fiery" in nature. Human suffering can damage this layer and lead to volcanic activity. These volcanos are a result of uncontrolled emotions of man, especially greed and hate. The type of energy portrayed by the Dragon, Ballrog in the movie, "Lord of the Rings" can be found here.
7. The next or 7th layer of the earth is the Mirroring Earth. It is given this name because they reflect the opposite of all phenomena. Colors are going to appear as the complementary form while even moral impulses, good or bad will be in the opposite form.

8. Splintering Earth is the name of the eighth layer as all living entities here are splintered into multiple copies of the original. This layer is also the source of black magic. Here, all good qualities are transformed into their opposites, which makes this layer an origin of all evil.
9. The 9th level, the earth core is where the utmost evil might be found. Here lies the deepest origin of Black magic. This layer resembles both the human brain and the human heart. It contains both the Demonic "I", the lower "I "as well as the possibilities of the higher "I"s.

The four layers, 6th – 9th are the most evil parts of the earth.
The 9th level is of great interest in regarding these connections. In our human body this is where we, in a way, leave the physical earth, and enter the Spiritual realm (the four levels of the "I", level 9 – 10 - 11 and 12. The 9th level is actually not part of the earth, but part of the cosmos. However, the 9th level is representing the lower "I", and as such this layer is also part of these evil layers.
According to my own spiritual investigations, there are 3 more layers of the internal earth. These three layers together with the 9th layer resemble the etheric layers of the internal heart of the human being. In the human heart, we can develop the higher self, the cosmic consciousness, as well as the Christ consciousness. The development of the last three last layers is evolutionary models for future development. The seeds of these three layers were put there by Christ himself on the 4th of April, in the year 33 following the crucifixion at Golgotha, after which he descended through the earth, through all the layers.
Reaching the 9th layer, the level of ultimate evil, he placed the seeds of a future heart, a heart to be created by the actions of the human race, in correlation with the creation of the three higher selves within the heart of the human being.

These same layers are in the earth. The 10th layer, the layer of the human "I" as a possibility for the future world, The 11th layer, the layer of the human higher "I" as a possibility for the future world, and the 12th layer, the layer of the Christ consciousness, the Christ "I" as a possibility for the future world.

Demonic powers influence us especially from the 6th and the 9th layer, and vice versa. If we are overpowered by greed and hate, the fire earth will rebel in volcanic eruptions and/or quakes. These influencing powers can only be counteracted through the strength of our higher I´s, and are in many ways equal to the effect of the higher "I´s" on Earth-Radiation as described as part of our karma. Listed below is a table summarizing the relationships of the 12 layers of the body and the 12 layers of the earth to the influences of the demonic realms.

	The layers of the body (according to Thoresen)	**The layers of the earth (according to Steiner)**
1st layer	The Astral sheath of the body	The physical earth
2nd layer	The Astral and the Physical/Material body	Fluid earth, high pressure, expansion
3rd layer	The Physical/Material body. If the physical is turned into Spirit, it shows the opposite. If a Spiritual entity points to one	*Damp (or air) earth.* Here the substances are in a damp state, this layer is full of life. This layer wants to expand even more than the 2nd layer. It is in close connection to passions in the human and the animal world, and the entire level is filled with

	direction, it means the other way.[61]	living streams consisting of strong passions. One peculiarity though, is that here all the emotions get changed into their opposite, love into hate and so on. Typical Luciferic actions.
4th layer	The Parasitic bodies within our Physical/Material body and alien physical bodies (bacteria) that we use to digest foodstuffs. Alien bodies also exchange DNA with us, as they are the source of physical development.	Water earth or form-earth. Here all substances are in an astral form. The astral form is the negative of the material form, just as in Devachan. These astral forms are the source of our astral development.
5th layer	I The Etheric body, warmth-ether (infra-red). Also the scars of the body, both physical and mental that have come from life's experiences of living in the warmth.	Fruit earth where everything is pure life. Everything is living here. This is the "blue-print" of all life, but in an inversed form.

---

[61] See further description of this phenomenon in my book "The forgotten mysteries of Atlantis" published on Amazon in 2015 - 2017.

6th layer	II The Etheric body, light-ether (blue = Ahriman, Red = Lucifer) Also the scars of the body, both physical and mental that have come from life, from living in the light.	Fire earth, which is in direct contact to human emotions, especially "fiery" emotions. Human suffering will upset this layer and lead to volcanic activity. "Dragon-energies" can be found here. Ballrog. Related to the magnetic field of the earth, and by such to Lucifer and earthquakes.
7th layer	III The Etheric body, Chemical-ether (Ultra-Violet). Also the scars of the body, both physical and mental that have come from life, from living in sounds and/or substances.	Mirroring earth or reflecting earth. Here are all the natural forces and laws found (all the laws used within physics), but in their opposite. All moral impulses are here changed into their opposite. All colours appear in their complementary colour (all ethers are here changed into their opposite).
8th layer	IV The Etheric body, Life-ether (Green). Also the scars of the body, both physical and mental that have come from	Splintering earth (layer of the numbers according to Pythagoras). All living entities are here splintered into multiple "copies" of the original.

		life, from living in the life-forces.	Source of black magic. All good qualities are here transformed into the opposite (= 7th layer). Origin of all evil in the world.
9th layer		The Demonic "I", the lower "I". The lower passions that we are aware of. Ill will.	The core of the earth. Here is the origin of Black magic. This layer resembles both the human brain and the human heart. It contains the Demonic "I", the lower "I"
10th layer		The "I", the ego, egoism. The "normal" self.	**(The 10th – 11th – 12th layer of the earth are according to Thoresen, not Steiner)** The "I", the ego, egoism, which may be transformed through the development of man into a good form of the "I".
11th layer		The higher "I", idealism. What we call the superego.	**(The 10th – 11th – 12th layer of the earth are according to Thoresen, not Steiner)** The higher "I", idealism which may be transformed through the development of man into a good form of the "I".

12th layer	The Christ "I", the Divine Consciousness, Christ-Consciousness.	**(The 10th – 11th – 12th layer of the earth are according to Thoresen, not Steiner)** The Christ "I", the divine consciousness, Christ-Consciousness that may be transformed through the development of man into a good and angelic form of the "I" (which may lift humans to the 10th hierarchy of angels).

Comparison of the 8th layer of the earth to the 8th layer of the body.

In the earth, the center of evil where Ahriman resides, is in both the 6th and the 8th layer. The 9th layer Rudolf Steiner describes as the core of the Earth. This core is like the human heart, housing egoistic feelings. As the heart is the hope of humanity, the growing power of the higher selves reside there, and will in the future become the 10th, 11th and 12th layer, expressing Christ-Consciousness. The 8th layer, however, will remain in close connection, with the 8th sphere. This 8th sphere will, in the future, branch off as the material earth and cannot develop together with the rest of the Spiritualizing earth and ascending humanity.

In the body, this 8th layer is also the center of evil, where the obstacles to therapy can be found. In the technique called neural therapy, it is recognized that certain scars can block the effectiveness of certain etheric modalities especially acupuncture.

The Demons relationships to our Auras

The "Spiritual Ahrimanic radiation" from the deeper layers of the earth enters both the weakened organs and organic processes, but also the weakened astral sheets that surround and protect our body

Weaknesses in any of the 3 Auras create holes or a passageway for demons. The luciferic Demons may enter mainly through the astral Aura, and the azuric demons may enter mainly through the Spiritual Aura. In addition, these weak spots can be created by the use of drugs (see addendum). Such weaknesses or passageways are also the cause of hypersensitive individuals. Spirits, and radiation of all kinds, including electromagnetic or Spiritual in origin, can easily influence these patients.

Sounds or other sensory influences may also influence us through auric weaknesses. In these subjects, skin may react as if sunburned, or radiated. The rays of the sun are in fact Spirits or Demons. As I mentioned earlier, electrical radiation comes from ahrimanic demons, while magnetic radiation comes from those of a luciferic origin. However, the worst effects come from the radiation of a combination of both demons, that of electromagnetic radiation. Finally, nuclear radiation is generated by Azuric demons.

Depending on the susceptible Aura, different Demons may enter. They then create disease for the person in question, and for all beings connected to that person. This includes the family, animals and even the trees and plants within the vicinity of the possessed individual.

Chapter 13:

Demons and Disease

The origins of ahrimanic and luciferic Demons.

According to Rudolf Steiner Lucifer has reached a higher state than man and is therefore considered a super-sensible being. The reason for this is that he is a spirit that has detached himself from the Spiritual hosts of heaven after the separation of the sun.

Ahriman[62] is also a higher super-sensible being, having already broken away before the separation of the sun and therefore is an embodiment of a different power. Ahriman opposes every creation with a negative counter-creation. His place of residence is the underworld, from which he brings darkness, death and mischief to the material world. Through Ahriman's work, man's insight into the spiritual is dulled, so that he only sees the physical realm. Matter is the kingdom of Ahriman where he brings the forces of death. Ahriman seduces man with lies which become germs of disease in later incarnations. He is the master of the intellect.

Lucifer brought man under the influence of the powers connected with air and water only, whereas it was Ahriman who has subjected man to the influence of far more deadly powers. The civilizations immediately to come will see the appearance of many things connected with Ahriman's influence. These influences involve powers of a much lower nature than those of Lucifer.

---

[62] Ahriman can be redeemed when he finds his essence in the mirror of human thought. "The salvation of Ahriman is through thought." As a defense against ahrimanic attacks, think about the first and eighth chapter of the Gospel of John (Lit.: GA 266c, p. 168)

Lucifer's influences can never become as evil as the influences of Ahriman.

The Role of Demons in Destructive Energy and Cancer

Destructive energy vs Cancer

In pulse-diagnosis occasionally we will find a pulse that actually can feel painful to the physician who is examining the patient. This is a reflection of a destructive energy that is present in the meridian. On palpation of the pulse, one gets a very distinct feeling. It is as if a pain travels from the pulse of the patient into our own body. This is called *"destructive energy"*. I have discovered that this is a result of the luciferic doppelgänger taking a hold of the ahrimanic doppelgänger as opposed to cancer where the ahrimanic doppelgänger takes hold of the luciferic doppelgänger.

A good example of the treatments regarding cancer is in the following case. A dog came to me that had been diagnosed with rectal cancer and had been treated without effect. The local veterinarian wanted to euthanize the dog, but the owner wanted to give the dog one last chance. When the dog and owner came to my home it was obvious that the nature of the illness was quite serious. The anus was swollen to the size of a large grapefruit, and partially ulcerated. The case was dire and any ordinary treatment would be useless. I decided to turn my intention and gaze in to the Demon world. There I saw an ugly looking Demon standing directly in front of the cancer. As the owner had been living with the North American Indians and believed in Demons, I told her what I had seen. She wanted me to "take the ugly Demon away" I carefully explained to her that if I did what she asked it would just be translocated only to harm another victim. This is described in the Bible: if a Demon is forced to leave a victim it hovers around for a while and then comes back to the original victim or to another entity. In doing so it might find a way to increase in strength or even enlist the help of other demons. The only way to really heal the disease is to transform the Demon. The only way to do this is through love and understanding and the light of the Christ. She immediately understood and accepted what I had told her.

I then put my hand over the Demon, and started to feel his pain, suffering, and anger, and forgave him in the name of Christ. His fierce look became milder and he withdrew to his own sphere. I asked the owner of the dog to keep me updated on his condition. The next day all of the cancer seemed to have disappeared. The swelling was down and the lymphatic circulation improved. All that remained was loose skin. However, the owner called me from her home and told me that some hours later the swelling started to come back.

While still in my own home, I addressed the Demon through focus and intention in an attempt to perform long distance healing. I saw the Demon before my inner eye hurting the dog. I repeated 3 times to the Demon: "Light in Christ". Then, after 30 minutes, I called up the dog owner and asked how it was. She told me that within a half an hour, the dog was totally normal.

In summation:

It is important to respect demons. They also have their own life and destiny. Demons *want* to be Transformed into the light. Although many fear the transformation and try to avoid it, Demons are trapped and *want* to become free. So, if we see, hear or feel demons, we need to understand that the mere sensing of them gives us some power over them. However, only Christ and the Christ-Consciousness has the power to free Demons

Chapter 14:

The Detection and Prevention of the demon-feeding effect of Earth-Radiation

In ancient times, people knew that there were innumerable entities, in the form of Elementals, within the Earth. These entities were usually considered harmful to humans and animals. As the time of enlightenment dawned in the 1500's, we stopped believing in these Elemental Beings and the mysterious forces that are associated with them. The pathological radiation coming from the earth is now explained as being electro-magnetic (sic). Such radiation is commonly known to be potentially pathological to all life forms. This is especially true in EMFs found under high voltage lines and from the emanations of cell phones. However, part of the problem in understanding the existence of "spiritual radiation" is that devices made for the detection of electro-magnetic radiation are only able to detect a minor part of all existing radiation. However, there are sensitive people, dowsers and clairvoyants who are capable of sensing and mapping these subtle force fields. Sadly, because they are the only ones possessing such skills, this led to the faulty conclusion that dowsers were finding radiation that did not exist. Now, in the modern age, my hope is that we find a way to acknowledge that the physical world is a manifestation of the Spiritual World. We need to understand that all radiation is related to Spiritual Beings, Elementals and Demons, as did those before us who strived to shield themselves from this Demonic radiation.

Tracing noxious radiation.

Four important methods are used to trace noxious radiation: these are listed below:
1. Divining instruments.
2. Technical instruments to detect electromagnetic distortions.
3. Bioassays: the use of living organisms such as mice, fish, insects or plants by observing their autonomic nervous system reactions as well growth and well-being while under the influence of noxious radiation.
4. Sensitivity and/or clairvoyance, which is necessary for tracing all Spiritual radiation or influences.

Divining instruments.

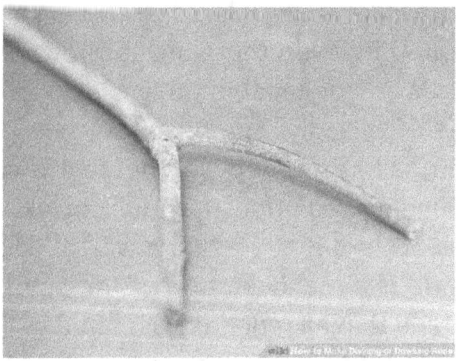

As recorded over eons of time, one can find noxious zones by dowsing, or divining. The dowser holds a divining rod (Y-stick), or other divining instruments such as a pendulum, rubbing pad, angle irons, etc. in the hands, and when the body's autonomic system senses a noxious influence, it increases muscle spasm. This causes the divining instrument to move or behave differently, thus indicating the location of the noxious radiation. However, the explanation that the body's autonomic system senses a noxious influence and reacts, is for me suspect. I sincerely believe that there are far stronger and unknown Spiritual forces working within Earth-Radiation that dictates the movement of such detection devices.

Technical equipment to detect electromagnetic distortions

One method is the use of a simple radio. If a transistor radio with its antenna extended, is tuned to "white noise ", that noise can change when the researcher moves over a zone that is distorted by Earth-Radiation. Other conventional methods, include electronic measuring equipment, such as a sensitive magnetometer that can also register the more physical types of Earth-Radiation, and yield more objective data than employing divining rods. Although the latter may prove impractical as a simple and accurate methodology, it has its merits in demonstrating that these radioactive emissions can be hazardous to our overall health.

German experiments on several hundred students in the time between the two World Wars showed how some people reacted immediately when exposed to Earth-Radiation. In these "noxious zones", such symptoms as malaise, vertigo and blurred vision were recorded. For example, blood pressure readings would change by as much as 20 to 30 points while traversing these zones. The dowsing reaction is proposed to be transmitted via the parasympathetic autonomic nervous system. This involuntary response controls respiration, heart rate, blood pressure, digestion and other organ functions. Therefore, measuring blood pressure and heart rate can show the changes that occur when a sensitive subject is placed over a noxious field[63]. Employing such

---

[63] Rupert Sheldrake: *A New Science of Life: The Hypothesis of Morphic Resonance* (1981) proposed that through "morphic resonance", various perceived phenomena, particularly biological ones, become more probable the more often

changes induced by the parasympathetic nervous system, we can then demonstrate the adverse effects of geopathic radiation. The problem lies in the fact that such instrumentation does not differentiate qualitatively between Earth-Radiation that causes disease and Earth-Radiation that is harmless. Also, they are unable to detect the most important Radiation, namely the Spiritual Earth-Radiation from the deep layers of the earth.

Skilled dowsers however, acknowledging the Spiritual side of Earth-Radiation, do have this ability as an innate reaction, regarding both the electromagnetic and the Spiritual aspects of this force.

Tracing noxious influences by bioassay using living organisms

As mentioned above, we have seen through the dowsing reaction induced by the autonomic nervous system, we can observe changes in subjects exposed to the adverse effects of geopathic radiation. This research has shown that influences of this nature adversely affect he immunity, growth and other parameters of health in plants, humans and animals. This phenomenon has been confirmed by the work of Peter Tompkins and Christopher Bird, authors of "The Secret Life of Plants". In this book, they discuss the effect Geopathic Radiation on the growth rate of hedges, plants and fruit trees.

Tracing or finding pathologic radiation through sensitivity and/or clairvoyance.

This method directly addresses the spiritual understanding of earth and exemplifies the true origins of radiation as energy generated from the spirit world. It can be performed in several

---

they occur, and that biological growth and behavior thus become guided into patterns laid down by previous similar events.

ways, but all ways require that we have entered the spiritual world through dividing our thinking, feeling and willing. These techniques include Nogiér's pulse diagnosis as performed in the field of auricular acupuncture (see part one of this trilogy) or by developing our spiritual senses such as our "spiritual eye", "spiritual nose", or "spiritual ear" as described in the third part of this book.

The spiritual foundation of earth radiation is the pathological expression of ahrimanic beings. The seeds of this pathological foundation including the effect of deeds performed before the existence of the human race (the deeds of the Brownies[64]), and the malevolent actions of human beings (murder, lying) after they were created.

Finding the Spiritual radiation from past sins or ahrimanic beings in the deeper layers of the earth is only possible through clairvoyance and Spiritual sensitivity. Since these causations are purely spiritual in nature, they can only be dealt with by spiritual means.

It is only by loving and forgiving past ill deeds, preferably in the name of Christ, can such radiation permanently be dissolved (much the same as dissolving the ahrimanic and the luciferic demons through the Middle/Christ-Point treated with Christ-Consciousness).

Modern scientists have repeatedly commented that if it really is radiation, it should be detectable through modern detection devices. Of course, some "radiation" of cosmic and earthly origin is detectable, however, that is of electromagnetic origin. This kind of radiation is not what we are referring to. We need to stop thinking of "earth" radiation as "radiation" understood by modern

---

[64] **The "Brownies"** are Elemental Beings found in a number of places in nature. They have no connections to humans but stay within themselves. They are **very** old and are possibly created by the deeds of former human races like the Neanderthals. They form communities with their own infrastructure, have no clothes, are small and hairy, and speak little. I have experienced seeing two colonies of these creatures.

scientists, and perhaps develop better nomenclature for this spiritual force.

A Unique Method to Diagnose Positional "Demonic Earth-Radiation" toxicity.

The noxious influence of Lay lines of geopathic radiation are dependent on their direction relative to the patient. I have developed a simple method that can detect a positional influence of Earth-Radiation. Patients that do not react to treatment might be under such constant influence, especially with regards to direction of sleep. We can use this method to find out, in case there really is such an influence, at what angle the line of Earth-Radiation hits the body. In this way, we can determine in what direction to move the animal or bed to avoid the pathological influence.

To obtain this information, we need a square, 5x5 cm piece of transparent plastic. The figure illustrated below is then drawn on this sheet.

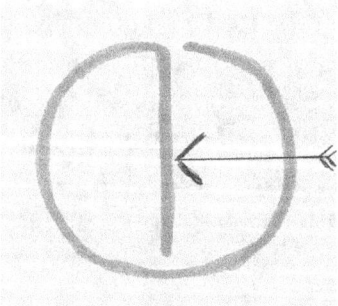

The plastic sheet is held in front of the ear of the patient, while we carefully control the pulse of Nogiér (RAC – VAS)[65]. We then slowly turn the plastic sheet around 360^0. At certain angles, there will be a distinct RAC/VAS. This reaction indicates that the patient is under the influence of pathological Earth-Radiation as the ear carries the memory of this influence in the ear.

At which angle this radiation hits the body can be calculated in the following way:

- The ear resembles the body itself, with the lobe as the head and the top of the ear as the legs.
- The RAC/VAS occurs when the straight line in the drawing creates an angle of 90^0 with the imprinted radiation.
- If the RAC/VAS occurs as indicated in the diagram below, it will mean that the radiation crosses or hits the body 90^0 to the longitudinal axis (to the median plane).
- If the patient then sleeps with the head to the north and the feet to the south, then the radiation line will go east-west or west-east.
- Then we know that the Organ-Systems in danger are either the Lungs or the Liver (see table below).
- Then the patient will have to move the bed further towards the head or the feet. If he moves the bed to the side, he will not avoid the radiation.

---

[65] **RAC / VAS** The pulse reaction, called the RAC or VAS by Nogiér, is an essential part of a thorough examination in auriculomedicine (as in "controlled AP" as well). This pulse response is a reflex from the skin to the heart or arterial blood circulation. Stimulation of the skin over a reactive area, a point or a weak structure activates an autonomic reaction or recognition that induces a special VAS Pulse reaction. The VAS-reaction may be found anywhere at an artery.

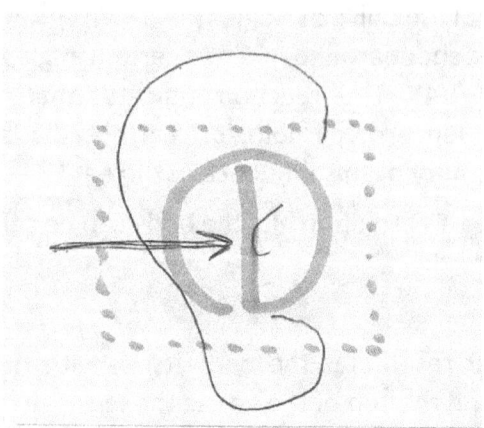

How to use this knowledge to treat patients

We have to keep in mind, if we are to use this knowledge; the direction of the electromagnetic or spiritual radiation decides which Organ-System it will affect. If the radiation is excessive It will cause damage. The associations of direction to organ systems are shown in the chart below:

From north	KI
	BL
From south	HT, PC,
	SI, TH
From west	LU
	LI
From east	LV
	GB

Now we can determine the Organ-System to stimulate using the determined direction of the radiation. We may then treat the organ in question with herbs or acupuncture. Of course, the patient should also be removed from the radiation. However, I have found that the radiation often follows the sick person.

Example

Dr. Georg Bentze, my acupuncture teacher, was once hired by the Oslo prison authorities to help some of the prisoners feel more comfortable and to induce a better sleep. He began by mapping out all the lines of Earth-Radiation under the beds of the prisoners. He noticed that there were a stronger and a greater amount of lines than usual. He supervised moving all the beds of the prisoners, and by the following night they slept better, felt more relaxed and demonstrated a greater enjoyment of life. The administrator of the prison was satisfied.

When he returned one month later to access the situation, he found, to his great surprise, that all the radiation lines had changed. They had followed the beds to their new positions, and now the situation was once again as it had been before. Dr. Bentze was unsure as to how to deal with or explain this phenomenon. The prison authorities discarded the entire experiment as its effect on the prisoners was not sustainable. This is a common misinterpretation among most. This is due to the fact that does not understand spiritual phenomena. I now understand that these lines were actually represented Demonic beings, created by the life and behavior of the prisoners themselves. They belong to the karmic grid that each person carries. That is why I no longer believe in isolating or shielding houses or beds from radiation. The only way to be free of the Demonic radiation is to acknowledge the origin, ask for forgiveness, and change one's life. The radiation is a part of ourselves and must be loved and respected.

The knowledge about the direction of radiation was known in ancient times by those who worked with animals and agriculture.

Today, this knowledge is largely forgotten, or disparaged as pseudoscience. This is a great mistake.

A little radiation, however, will actually stimulate our etheric energy, and there is always some radiation everywhere (there is always a presence of Elemental Beings which we need). Standing or sleeping with the head towards a special direction, *unless a Demonic Earth-Radiation also happens to come from that direction*, will be beneficial to the Organ-System in question.

For example, if a cow is standing with its head (the head being the receiver of cosmic radiation) towards north, the cow will receive energy that stimulates the kidneys. If a horse is standing with its head towards east, the energy will stimulate the liver. Farmers in Austria knew this, and their old tradition was to let the cows stand with the heads towards north, and horses towards east which are their respective inherit deficiencies.

This knowledge may also be used therapeutically. If a patient has problems with an Organ-System, it will be beneficial to stand or lay with the head in the stimulating direction of the Organ-System in question.

Medieval Spiritual ways of protection

Many Spiritual methods of how to protect oneself from demonic influences are described in the literature derived from Medieval times. Some texts recommend Imagining oneself to be a fully armored knight, holding a huge long sword. One is to then stand against the north and touch the ground with the tip of the sword. Where the tip touches the ground, a flame will light up. Then slowly turn towards west and continue turning, south, east and back to north again, thus creating a full circle around oneself using the tip of the sword. When the circle is finished, a flaming circle will form where the circular tracing was etched. Within this enflamed circle one will be protected for 12 hours before the procedure needs to be reapplied. Other forms of visualization include standing inside a circle of mirrors, reflecting back all radiation coming in. This procedure will afford protection for 24 hours.[66]

As described in the introduction of this part of the trilogy, as a veterinarian in Bodø, Northern Norway, I was treating a cow with milk-fever who suddenly died. Every two weeks the same experience occurred. After realizing that the cause of these three deaths was black magic cast by a neighbor, I performed a ritual, protecting the barn from evil. I did this by going around the entire structure imagining that I was a knight in shining armor, encircling the area with my sword. Where the sword touched the ground flames shot up, and after completing the circle, the barn and the cows were protected by a wall of fire. After that no more cows died.

The phenomenon of smoke[67] as a protection against Demons

The use of smoke in religious connections is as old as humanity itself. In the Old Testament, it is told that both Cain and Abel made burning sacrifices to God, and the way that the smoke behaved, indicated whether or not God accepted their offerings. Abel's smoke rose upwards into the air, whilst the smoke from Cain's offering stayed close to the earth. My understanding of this is that Abel's smoke was able to drive away the earth-bound Spirits and open his mind to God. Cain on the other hand was destined to work with the earth, to struggle his way through the earthly domain and as such, also fight both the luciferic and the ahrimanic demons.

---

[66] Many more methods are described in the book "Clavicula Salomonis".

[67] I have often wondered why the use of "MOXA" within acupuncture treatment is so effective. When the moxa is burned it gives off quite much smoke. This smoke may be causes the demonic entities to translocate.

A combination of smoke and smell is essential for the effect of the procedure, even though the smoke seems to be the most important part of the two. I have always felt the peace and quiet that descends after making a campfire. Once the campfire is lit and the smoke wafts and is smelled amongst the trees, it feels is if the camp has become a home. I feel peaceful as the fire burns. For me, if feels as if the evil Spirits are driven away and the good Spirits are called upon.

In many different religious ceremonies dedicated to the gods, incense is often used around the alter to keep the Demons away and possibly transform them. The American Indians often burn white sage to cleanse the body before ritual ceremonies.

A few years ago, my left retina suffered from a detachment, which required surgery. During my convalescence, in my weakened state, I could feel a closing in of the ahrimanic and luciferic demons into my left orbit. After I made a fire in the fireplace of my living room, I suddenly felt a strong urge to close the pipe, and let the room fill with smoke. The rest of the day I felt very well, despite the unpleasant aroma. However, the next day my misery returned. Suddenly had an enlightening inspiration regarding the smoke. I went to fetch a piece of "san-paulo-wood" used for incense burning, and set fire to it. When I blew out the flame, the room was filled with the smoke of the incense. As I waved the smoking piece around me, I immediately felt the luciferic and the ahrimanic Demons of the disease loosen their grip. This was, for me, a huge revelation.

I once was acquainted with a German doctor who specialized in diagnosing diseases with his etheric sense of smell. His treatment was to then apply specific Etheric oils or fragrances to the bedclothes of his patients. In this way, he could counteract the smell of the disease. The smell of the oils drove the Demons away. Both the application of smoke and etheric oils are examples of driving the "disease-Demons" out of the body. However, the problem lies the fact that the demons are only translocated with these methods and made available to harm the next unsuspecting host.

At a Seattle acupuncture meeting, four Indian attendees asked me to participate in the Indian ceremony of smoking a peace-pipe. We were sitting in a circle, sending the pipe around. The tobacco used was not a hallucinogen and consisted only of ordinary plants and tobacco. However, the smoke had an etheric effect on the room. The atmosphere became markedly lighter. The chief Indian called for the good spirits of the earth and asked the demonic spirits to depart. Then, in the middle of the ceremony the door to the room opened, and a traditionally dressed Indian entered. I was amazed by his presence, as he wore the full feather-ornamented traditional dress. This seemed rather odd to me especially in the 14th floor of a posh Settle high rise. He then closed the door and stood for a while looking at our circle. I asked the Indian beside me what he was doing here. With astonishment he asked me; "Do you see him? If so you are the first white man ever to see him". The smoke and the ritual had cleared the room of ahrimanic and evil Spirits allowing the appearance of this old shaman. In all cultures and even in orthodox services, the burning of incense has been used to clear away evil Spirits and Demons.

My entire life I wondered why people enjoyed smoking. Now I understand its appeal. The pleasure is in a moment, to be free of demons. Sadly, like all addictive substances, that moment never lasts, and as the law of attraction demands, there will be even more when the cigarette but is rubbed out.

The importance of Archangel Michael's fight against Demons.

The Archangel Michael[68], aside from Christ himself, is a demon's greatest adversary. He is the warrior Angel sent by God to help

---

[68] **Michael** ("who is like God") is an archangel in Judaism, Christianity and Islam. Roman Catholics, the Eastern Orthodox, Anglicans and Lutherans refer to him as "Saint Michael the Archangel" and also as "Saint Micheal". In the New Testament Michael leads God's armies against Satan's forces in the Book of

protect us from these entities. Michael stands beside Christ as the commander of all the legions of angels in their fight against these hordes of demons. There are many stories about how Michael, the Spiritual being of the rank of archangeloi, led the legions of angels in the great battle against Ahriman and Lucifer.

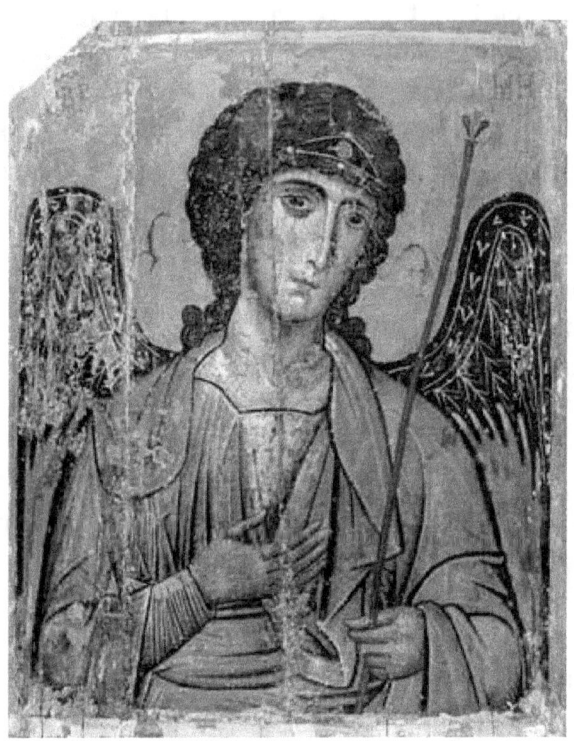

Revelation, where during the war in heaven he defeats Satan. In the Epistle of Jude, Michael is specifically referred to as "the archangel Michael". Christian sanctuaries to Michael appeared in the 4th century, when he was first seen as a healing angel, and then over time as a protector and the leader of the army of God against the forces of evil. By the 6th century, devotions to Archangel Michael were widespread both in the Eastern and Western Churches. Over time, teachings on Michael began to vary among Christian denominations.

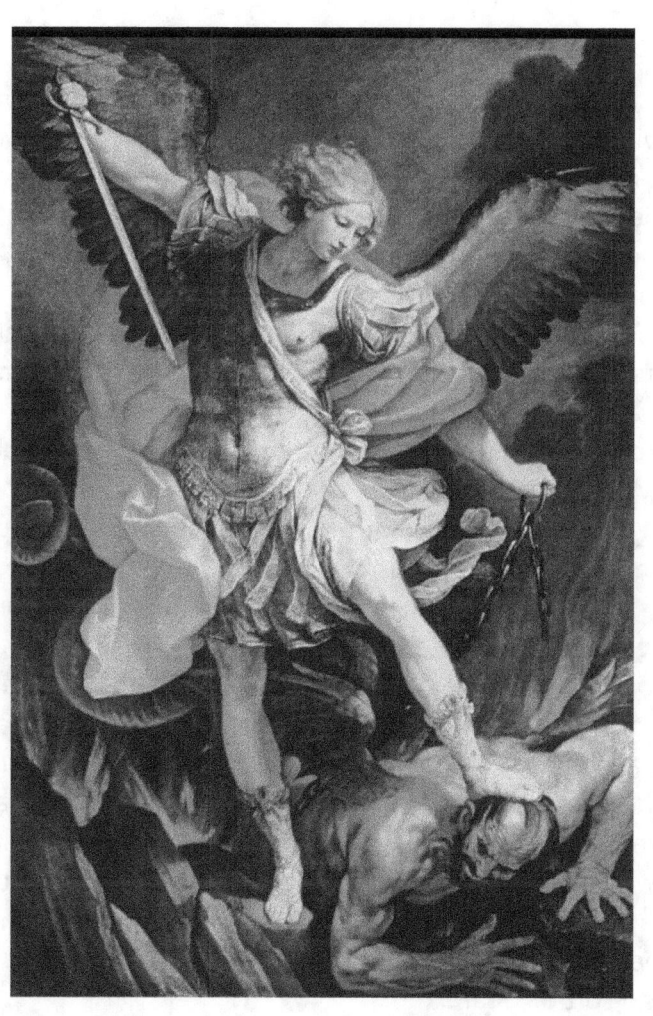

Medicinal plants in the use of treating demons.

For those with the ability to spiritually "see" demons in people and animals, they describe these entities as all having have a personal or individual look. In fact, the demons relating to a specific disease will look very similar yet vary slightly from person to person. For example, there are demons that accompany influenza and in such an epidemic these demons will be similar in appearance, as in a group of flu-demons, verses common-cold-demons.

In the same token, the Spirits of plants of the same family look alike but are not identical. It is also interesting to note, that while most of the flower spirits look quite attractive, this is not so with the medical plants. Plant-Spirits of poisonous and medical plants actually look quite frightening. In fact, the poisonous Plant-Spirits, at least for those plants that are medicinal, look very much like the demons that created the disease. As stated in the law of similars, plant-Spirits that look similar to the disease-bringing-Spirits can cure the related diseases.

Therefore, it is said that *"like cures like"*, just as Hahnemann, the father of homeopathy, postulated. In actuality, the healers of medieval times also observed that plants often carried a *"signature"* that resembled the disease they worked against. However, this *"signature-law"*[69] has even more significance for those who can see Spirits and Demons. This lot can "see" that the disease demons are actually supplanted by their twin counterpart as if the shock of being in the presence of something so similar creates a sort of "fear".

Many average healers who use this knowledge, but are unaware of such entities, have overlooked this deeper insight. Over time the significance of demonology regarding this Law has lost its meaning, and today the *"law of signature"* is presented as merely

---

[69] Signature-law: A medieval law in herbal medicine stating that the look of the plant will indicate against which disease it will be helpful.

coincidental. However, in earlier centuries, healers were quite aware that similar spirits frightened each other. That is why they made pictures or sculptures of small Demons on the corners of churches. They believed that these images would scare the real demons away.

In the plant world, this works in much the same way. We administer a medical plant to the patient, that carries the same spirit *(same appearance)* as the Demon that carries the disease. The plant-spirits, however, are not easily frightened by the disease-Spirits as humans. The plant-spirits are actually much braver than disease demons, and as such, can easily annihilate the disease.

The phenomenon of jolting (succusion)

In 1982, I participated in a three-day *Qigong* course with 70 other participants. An Asian instructor, a specialist in his field as well as a clairvoyant, instructed the course. For the first exercise, he asked us to stand in a specific Qigong-stance. He explained that this stance was to free oneself of any attached demons.

As directed, all participants stood in this somewhat unpleasant position. After a few minutes, the other participants began to tremble, shiver and groan. After a short time, the stance became more and more unpleasant. The groaning intensified as everyone began to shake, as if they were having an epileptic fit.

I was somewhat amazed and embarrassed to find that I was the only participant who was not trembling. I looked around, and felt totally alienated. I assumed that something must be wrong with me. I asked the instructor what I was doing wrong.

He told me that I was performing the stance correctly. Because this Qigong position was designed to expel demons attached to the body, this cleansing was what was causing the trembling. *"You"*, he continued, *"seem not to have any attached demons. You can stop performing the stance"* …… and so I did.

I noted later that a host's body may shiver, some less and some more, when my acupuncture treatment results in their expulsion. In the demon exorcism used by the Catholic church, there are many eye witness descriptions recounting how the body of the person from whom the demon is expelled always shivers and jolts. This phenomenon is also used in homeopathy when preparing a remedy. In this context, the technique is referred to as succession, as part of a procedure called potentization[70]. For many years I wondered why, when making the remedy, it had to be shaken so vigorously between each of the stages of potentization. After I began to *"see"* the elemental forces in medical plants as well as in diseases, I developed a deeper understanding of this procedure.

As stated earlier, the characteristics of the elemental beings within the remedy look very similar to the pathological being that causes the disease. This is the basis of the homeopathic law of "likes treat likes" homeopaths postulate that the "energy" of the substance translocates into the water when the dilution is shaken. It is my opinion, that this shaking enables the spirit of the healing plant to translocate into the remedy.

---

[70] Potentization: A process in which a substance is diluted and then vigorously shaken in a process called succession. IE: when making a 1x (1:9 ration of substance to water) plant remedy, place 10 grams of plant material into 90 grams of 30% alcohol, and steep for one week. Strain the mixture, keeping 10 grams of the liquid. Mix this with 90 grams of water. Finish by "shaking" the mixture by hitting the bottle against a surface.

Our best protection against demons

Unlike the old rituals of the past, today I have found better ways to protect ourselves. By connecting to the good forces, having greater knowledge, insight and consciousness regarding these benevolent energies we are enlisting the power of the Christ impulse. Listed below are some suggestions:

1. *Pray* to your guiding spirits, your angels.
2. *Do not fight* the adversaries. Trust in the good forces.
3. Try to *help and transform* the demon (love thy enemy).
4. *Knowledge* about the inhabitants and existence of the spiritual worlds, especially about the adversaries.
5. *Insight* into the workings and laws of the Spiritual worlds. These are very different from the laws of the physical world.
6. *Consciousness* about the presence of the spiritual worlds, especially the angelic world, but also of its demons.
7. A strong *"I"-function* (especially in the 10th, 11th and 12th layer of the heart, the Christ level). At this level, the Demons have no power at all.

Chapter 15:

The Hexagon: Spiritual Beings and drugs

Many people using drugs say that they encounter alien entities. Perhaps this could be one of the reasons it is believed that such entities are merely hallucinations of the drugs. In my opinion, this is an invalid conclusion.

I have discovered that psychotropic substances open portals into a *real* Spiritual world. Furthermore, these doorways, once opened, can be travelled both ways. This opening allows entities living in the spiritual world (both good and bad) to enter us, and for us to enter the spiritual realm.

Therefore, we need to be conscious enough to defend ourselves and keep our "I", free of such demonic forces. The entities that have our wellbeing at heart want us to develop as Spiritual Beings but wisely wait for our proper preparation.

All doorways to the spiritual worlds are "personal", and must be entered by a spiritually developed consciousness. In order to be clear about who and what it is we are dealing with, we must understand the spirit world, know its inhabitants and be able to protect ourselves should we meet such undesirable influences.

The knowledge that other dimensions are inhabited by entities is also very important when we evaluate, describe and understand the workings of psychotropic plants and hallucinogens, especially when the unsuspecting attempt to use these substances to enter the spiritual world.

Hallucinogenic Experience: Reality or Fantasy

The use of psychedelic substances may open a portal to an "alternate reality". In addition, this reality is the dimension referred to in Anthroposophy as the "Spiritual World". The second premise relates to the theory that the hexagonal structure of the benzene ring found in the majority of mind altering chemical compounds may act as a spiritual bridge. My final premise requires a deeper understanding of the teachings of Rudolf Steiner which implies that the spirit world contains domains which are both benevolent and harmful. For the observer, often the ability to discern the difference between these domains can be problematic.

The encounter of spiritual Beings while under the influence of Hallucinogens

As stated above, it is my experience that psychotropic substances can open doorways or portals into a real Spiritual world. In addition, this doorway, once opened, can be travelled both ways. Therefore, I believe, that if one makes the poor decision to ingest such substances, he/she should realize the dangers of the destructive influences that may cause harmful effects to the user. According to Anthroposophy, it is of paramount importance to keep our higher consciousness, or our "I", free of such entities in order to protect our overall health.

Therefore, if one makes the unwise choice of employing such harmful substances, they should at least understand that this leads to a false path toward the evil aspects of the spiritual world. Rudolf Steiner believed that protection from such entities must come from an understanding of how to balance the adversarial powers (Lucifer and Ahriman) using a Christ-Consciousness. A better solution, however, is to abstain from drugs of such nature entirely.

Hallucinogenic chemical effect on the human body

My biochemistry training was rich in the study of the existence of various naturally occurring hexagonal compounds. These six sided molecules are referred to as benzene rings. I also learned that substances containing a nitrogen atom, followed by two or three carbon-atoms and a Benzene-ring are present in most hallucinogenic substances. Therefore, I hypothesized that this hexagonal shape may provide a link to other-dimensional qualities. Depicted below are the molecular structures of some of the more important psychotropic substances used today.

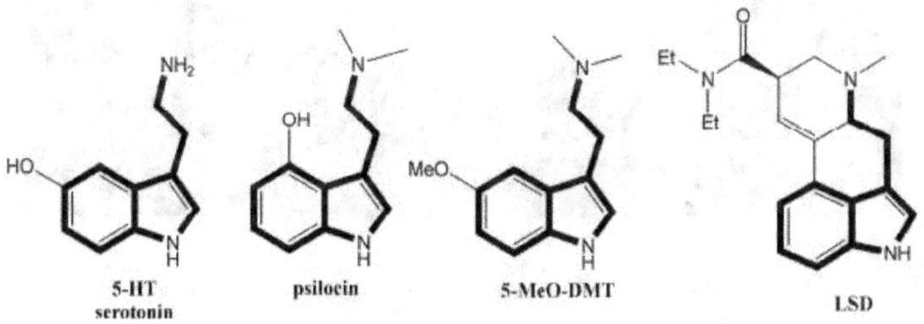

5-HT serotonin

psilocin

5-MeO-DMT

LSD

For example, Psilocybin (5-MeO-DMT) is a hallucinogenic compound that is similar to chemicals produced in the neurogenic part of the Pituitary gland. The most common psychedelic drug, LSD is also comprised of a similar chemical composition.
Rudolf Steiner illuminated the significance of this succession of atoms, in relation to the spiritual world:

> "But we must now go farther. I have placed two things side by side; on the one hand the carbon framework, wherein are manifested the workings of the highest spiritual essence which is accessible to us on Earth: the human Ego, or the cosmic spiritual Being which is working in the plants.

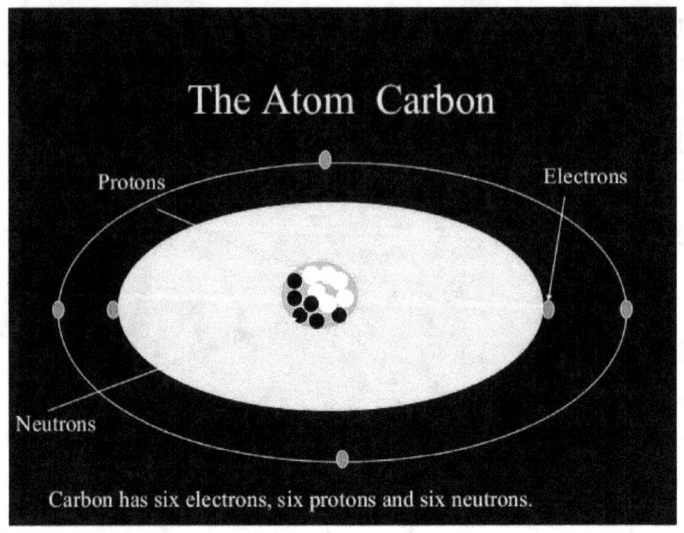

Observe the human process: we have the breathing before us the living oxygen as it occurs inside the human being, the living oxygen carrying the ether. And in the background we have the carbon-framework, which in the human being is in perpetual movement. These two must come together. The oxygen must somehow find its way along the paths mapped out by the framework. Wherever any line, or the like, is drawn by the carbon — by the spirit of the carbon — whether in man or anywhere in Nature there the ethereal oxygen-principle must somehow find its way. It must find access to the spiritual carbon-principle. Flow does it do so? Where is the mediator in this process?

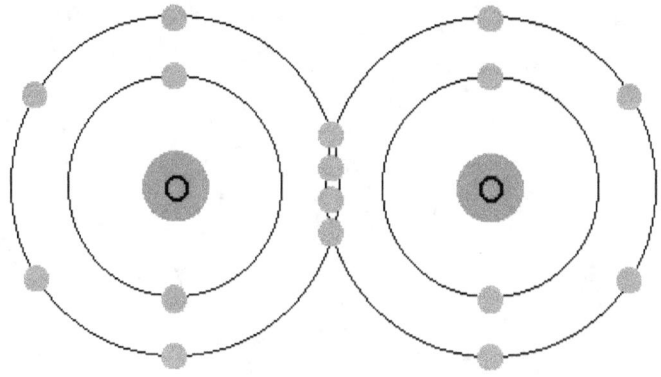

The mediator is none other than nitrogen. Nitrogen guides the life into the form or configuration, which is embodied in the carbon. Wherever nitrogen occurs, its task is to mediate between the life and the spiritual essence, which to begin with is in the carbon-nature. Everywhere — in the animal kingdom and in the plant and even in the Earth — the bridge between carbon and oxygen is built by nitrogen. And the spirituality which — once again with the help of sulphur is working thus in nitrogen, is that which we are wont to describe as the astral. It is the astral spirituality in the human astral body. It is the astral spirituality in the Earth's environment. For as you know, there too the astral is working — in the life of plants and animals, and so on.

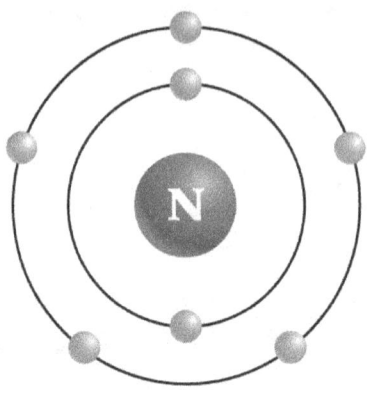

nitrogen

$^{14}_{7}N$

Thus, spiritually speaking we have the astral placed between the oxygen and the carbon, and this astral, impresses itself upon the physical by making use of nitrogen. Nitrogen enables it to work physically. Wherever nitrogen is, thither the astral extends. The ethereal principle of life would flow away everywhere like a cloud, it would take no account of the carbon-framework were it not for the nitrogen. The nitrogen has an immense power of attraction for the carbon-framework. Wherever the lines are traced and the paths mapped out in the carbon, thither the nitrogen carries the oxygen — thither the astral in the nitrogen drags the ethereal. Nitrogen is forever dragging the living to the spiritual principle. Therefore, in man, nitrogen is so essential to the life of the soul. For the soul itself is the mediator between the Spirit and the mere principle of life. Truly, this nitrogen is a most wonderful thing. If we could trace its paths in the human organism, we should perceive in it once more a complete human being. This "nitrogen-man" actually exists. If we could peal him out of the body he would be the finest ghost you could imagine. For the nitrogen-man imitates to perfection whatever is there in the solid human framework, while on the other hand it flows perpetually into the element of life."

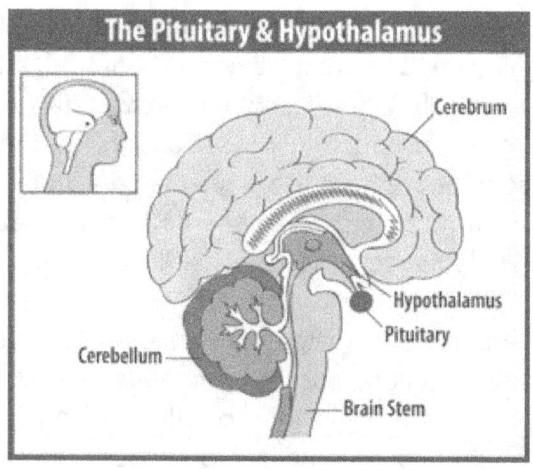

The Pituitary Gland

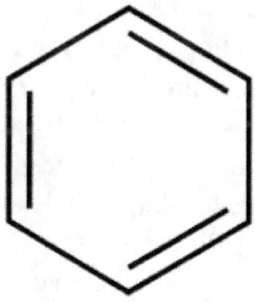

The Benzene-ring

In order to understand the effect these compounds have on how the individual perceives the spiritual world, we need to understand its inhabitants. As already mentioned, Steiner divided the malevolent forces into two fundamental archetypes. He often referred to these forces as demons.

The first archetype is referred to as Lucifer. The entities representing this impulse are usually very beautiful, attractive and often female-like. They are described throughout history and in many religious manuscripts. In Tantric Buddhism, they are often considered benign, and they help people to acquire knowledge and artistic inspiration. In the Tibetan 'Book of the dead' they are described as helping deceased spirits. Lucifer means the light-bearer, and as such, they emanate a strong blinding light. Although seemingly spiritual, they can often lead one astray. Folklore describes this confusion immediately after death. The soul is presented with two lights to follow toward the afterlife. One light is bright and blinding, the other soft and subtle. Most are tempted to choose the brighter Luciferic light. However, the better choice is to follow the soft light. The one that leads to Christ, the only path that will lead to salvation. When the Tibetan book of the dead was written, Christ had not yet appeared, therefore the Luciferic influence was the only one that could help with mankind's spiritual evolution.

Therefore, I suggest that hexagonal structures provide not only an opening to the spiritual world but also, that specific compounds provide access to specific aspects of this domain. For example, regions controlled by Luciferic influences are illuminated by the effect of LSD, DMT or Psilocybin. This is especially true for DMT, which is produced by the Pituitary gland. Rudolf Steiner describes this organ as highly spiritual and believes it is the remnant of our clairvoyant third eye or the 6th chakra.

Steiner also revealed that the spiritual world contains a region he called the "eighth sphere". In my experience, it can be entered by the ingestion of DMT. In this world, the inhabitants appear insect like. This becomes even more significant when one considers the hexagonal structure of the insect eye. In addition, insects have a tendency to construct hexagons, such as the honeycomb.

Studies have shown that at the moment of death, the Pituitary gland excretes a large amount of DMT. If one agrees that this compound is capable of opening a portal to the Luciferic world, this would explain the near-death experience of seeing a bright light. Although a possible source of comfort, as stated earlier, the brightest light presents the path toward Lucifer.

In my personal experience, I have found that ingesting a high dose of DMT can open a portal to the 8th sphere, a portal to the more malevolent influence of Ahriman. Steiner stresses that there is an oppositional relationship between the forces of Ahriman and Lucifer. This opposition represents a balance of power that minimizes the effect of either one on the soul of man. This might explain the beneficial effect of honey produced by the hexagonal structure of the hive. From an Anthroposophic medical viewpoint, the honey made by bees counteracts the sclerosing effect of Ahrimanic impulses. We may then understand the beneficial influence of Luciferic impulses through the bees that work for our health and balance.

The discovery of the Benzene-ring

How this structure was discovered yields interesting information regarding its possible Luciferic origin. Literature is filled with examples of Lucifer appearing as a snake or dragon. In relation to this finding, Friedrich August Kekulé, the German chemist who discovered the Benzene ring, wrote about two dreams he had at key moments of his work.

In his first dream, in 1865, he saw atoms dance around and link to one another. He awakened, and immediately began to sketch what he visualized. Later, he had another dream, in which he saw these atoms form themselves into strings, moving about in a snake-like fashion. This vision continued until the train of atoms formed into an image of a snake eating its own tail. This dream gave Kekulé the idea of the cyclic and hexagonal structure of benzene.

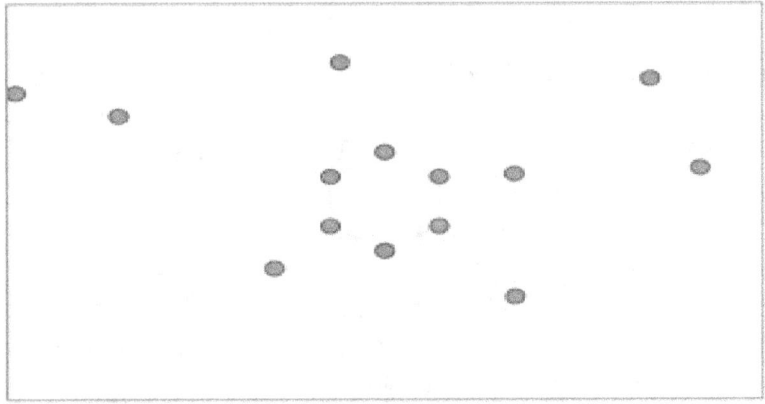

Figure 1: Six carbons have linked to form a chain.

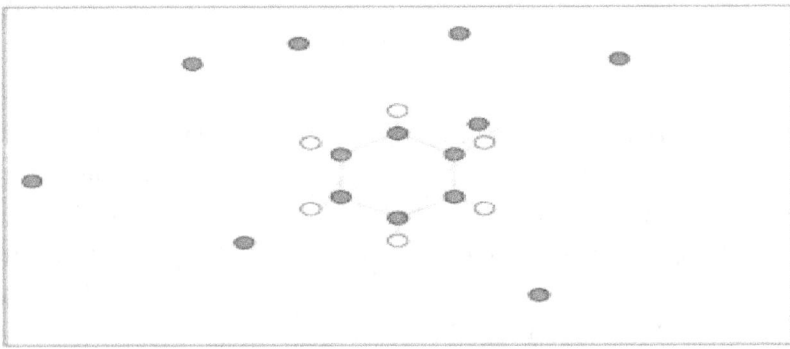

Figure 2: The chain has closed to form a hexagonal "ring."

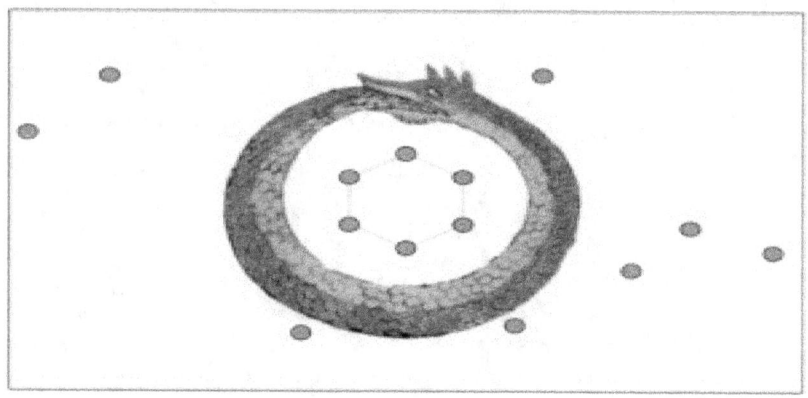

Figure 3: The ring is surrounded by a snake eating its own tail.

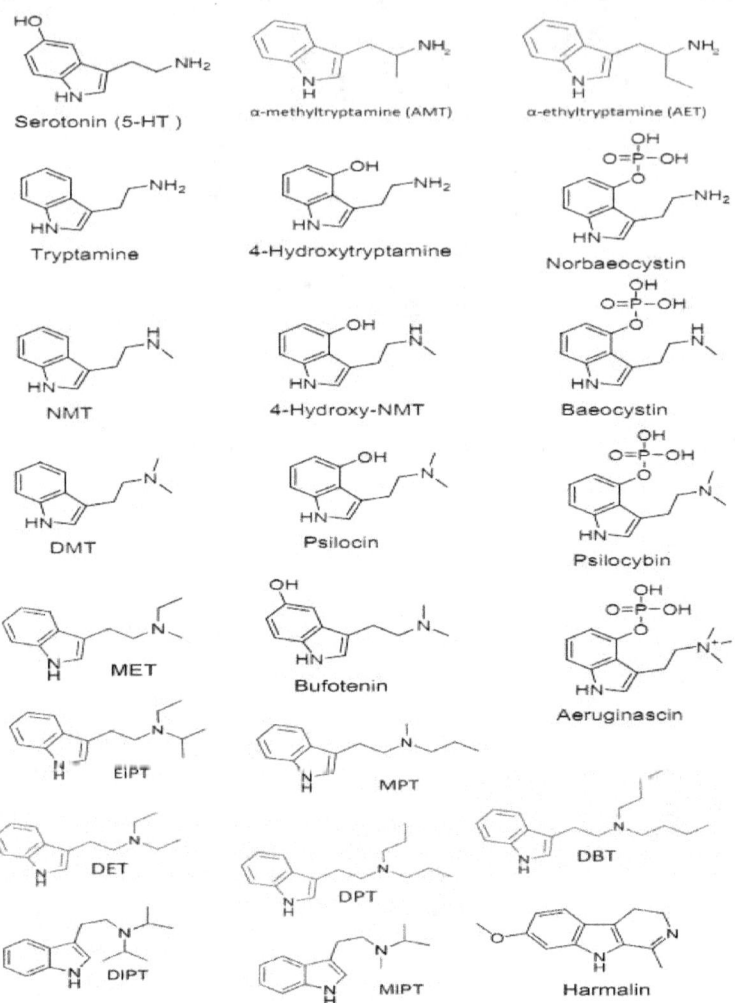

Some other hallucinogenic substances.

Examples of hexagonal portals in nature

An interesting example of the connection between hexagonal structures, Luciferic beings, and hallucinogenic properties is Fingal's Cave in Scotland. In ancient times, it was written that this cave was used for the initiation of the Druids. Later, it became famous as the source of inspiration for music composed by Felix Mendelssohn. In my opinion, Mendelssohn was influenced by the opening of a Luciferic portal related to the time of the year, the type of light that was illuminating the cave at the moment of his inspiration, and the hexagonal structures of this landmark.

A Scottish writer has suggested a new link between Felix Mendelssohn's famous composition the 'Hebrides Overture' and this landmark. This work was purposely finished on December 16th, 1830, the only day of the year the cave is fully illuminated by sunlight. Mendelssohn visited the cave in 1829 while on a tour of Scotland and completed his Hebrides Overture on December 16th of the following year.

A phenomenon has been frequently reported that one can hear profound musical performances while visiting this cave. I have personally experienced this music and was transposed into another realm of existence.

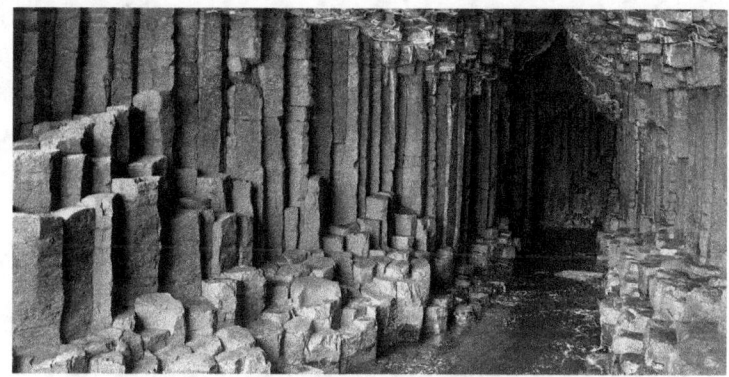

Fingal's Cave at Staffa where music may be heard

The same hexagonal structures can be found at another place in Scotland, at Giant's Causeway or footsteps.

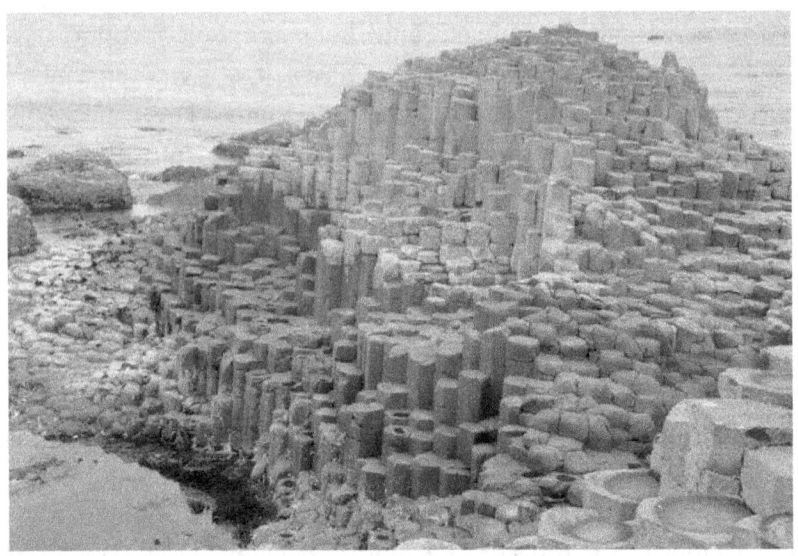

Giant's Causeway (footsteps) in Scotland

Don't Do Drugs: The danger of hallucinogens:

The danger of using hallucinogenic or psychotropic substances cannot be overstated. Not only for the obvious physical damage done to the human brain, But, more importantly, for the devastation that they can inflict upon the soul. The spiritual world must be approached with great knowledge and reverence. It is imperative that we don't open ourselves to the darker Spirits and allow them into our being. There is no rational for using such malevolent compounds. As Steiner has stated, there are no shortcuts in spiritual evolvement. Entering the spiritual world can only be mastered using the shield of a clear and present consciousness and going through the stages of initiation as described in this book.

Chapter 16:

The Dangers of Demons in the Use of Alternative Medicine

Dangers of homeopathy

It is my opinion, that complicated ritualistic procedures are often a cloak for the ability to siphon energy to darker forces. I have already discussed my opinion on this subject using the example of the ritualistic procedures found with the Reiki method. I suspect this same kind of ritualism has been injected into classical homeopathy. If the procedure of potentization is kept simple and "clean", the spirit of the mother tincture will be freed from the material substance and transferred to the water. However, in some instances, if this procedure has been unduly complicated, as in <u>double-dilution</u> LM prescribing, unwanted "openings" in the etheric might be created. Thus allowing a siphoning of portions of the homeopathic energy to the creator of the complex ritual.

This can also occur when potentization is done by machines (as in very high potencies). The use of an electrically operated device opens a portal to the Ahrimanic world

Dangers of acupuncture

The same dangers as described in homeopathy may arise within acupuncture or other reflexology procedures. If some influential "Guru" has described a complicated treatment to obtain an effect, I have found that the results may be linked to the originator of such procedures. I have also discovered that if ahrimanic or luciferic spirits have inspired the inventor, a link to the darker side is established.

The patient will of course feel cured and know nothing of these described connections, but the toll of the healing of that patient will be a strengthening of the dark side, and a connection established between the healer, the patient and the "dark world".

Mediums and Demons.

Unlike benevolent entities, demons do not have to respect the free will of their hosts. Rudolf Steiner is quite clear about the use of mediums. In his lectures [71]

> *"We can only know what the elementary beings are, the progeny of the Ahrimanic powers, when we enter into the world immediately bordering on our own. These beings manifest through mediums. They take possession of the mediums and in this way temporarily enter our world. If we contact them through a human medium only, we learn to know them in a world that should really be foreign to them; we do not know them in their true form. Spiritual revelations are undoubtedly transmitted, but it is impossible to understand them when they issue from a world to which they do not belong. The deceptive and highly hallucinogenic element in everything connected with mediumistic consciousness is explained by the fact that those who contact these beings have no understanding of their real nature. Now, because they enter the world in this way a unique destiny is reserved to these beings. The knowledge of the universe that I have described serves to enlarge our field of knowledge. When we enter the world of the dead, we traverse Demonic forests of poisonous plants like Colchicum autumnale, Digitalis Purpurea (Purple foxglove), Datura Stramonium (thorn-apple) and so on. The poisonous plants are moribund plants, species that are dying out, with no possibility of future development. In the future, they will*

---

[71] True and false paths in Spiritual investigations, lecture eight; "Potential aberrations in Spiritual investigation", given on the 9th of August 1924,

be replaced by other poisonous species. The poisonous species of today are already dying out in our epoch. The epoch of course is of long duration, but these poisonous plants have the seeds of death within them. And this will be the fate of all vegetation. When we survey the world of vegetation with this Spiritual vision we perceive forces of growth and development with a dynamic urge towards the future and a world that is dying and doomed to perish. And so it is with the beings that take possession of the mediums. They detach themselves from their companions, whose task is to carry over the present into a distant future. Through the agency of mediums they invade the world of the present, and are there caught up in the destiny of the Earth and sacrifice their future mission. In this way, they deprive man to a large extent of his future mission. And this is what faces us when we understand the real nature of mediumism, for mediumism implies that the future shall perish in order that the present may be very important. When therefore we attend a séance with insight into the real occult relationships and into the true nature of the Cosmos, we are at first astonished to find that the entire circle participating in a Spiritistic manifestation is seemingly surrounded by poisonous plants. Every Spiritualistic séance is surrounded in fact by a garden of poisonous plants which no longer bear the same aspect as in the kingdom of the dead, but which grow up around the Spiritualist circle, and from their fruits and flowers Demonic beings are seen to emerge. Such is the experience of the clairvoyant at a Spiritualistic séance. For the most part, he goes through a kind of cosmic thicket of poisonous plants that are activated from within and are part animal. Only by their forms do we recognize that they are poisonous plants. We learn from this how everything at work within this mediumistic form that ought to advance the course of human evolution and bear *fruit in the future is relegated to the present where it does not belong. In the present, it works to the detriment of humanity. Such is the inner mystery of mediumism, a mystery of which we shall learn more in the course of these lectures."[72]*

It has become more apparent to me, that the Ahrimanic Demons are very intelligent and translocate to avoid being seen or attacked. The classic séances as described above and as they are described by Rudolf Steiner in these lectures, are not at all performed today as they were a 100 years ago. Today the Demons have taken on the disguise of the modern world, and Mediums that are hysterical or half unconscious are rare. In fact, those encountered today seem to be totally conscious and intelligent people.

---

[72] http://wn.rsarchive.org/Lectures/GA243/English/RSP1969/19240819p01.html#sthash.Xbdprbb7.dpuf

Spiritual Medicine

Part Three

The Middle and the Group

"Where two or three are gathered"

The Faculty of Willing

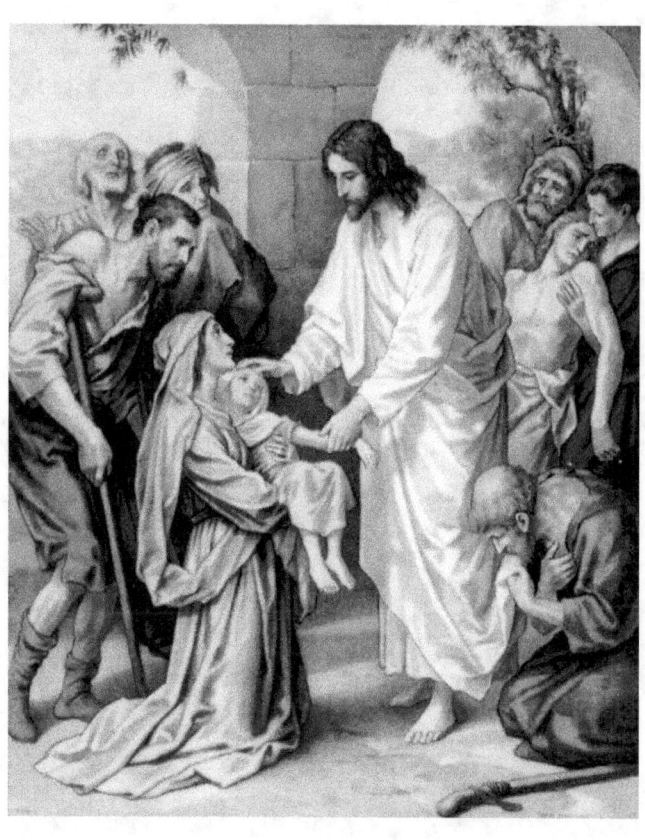

Chapter 17:

My Struggle with Cancer Treatment

My journey to self-discovery

Sometimes our greatest struggles guide us to our greatest achievements. For me, this struggle came with the treatment of cancer. The dilemma began with my use of acupuncture meridian therapy according to the five elements.[73] However, with time, I was guided toward spiritual medicine and, beyond this, the greater concept of treating humanity as a whole (the group).

My journey toward understanding the nature of cancer began in 1983. I realized, at that time, that cancer had to be treated differently from other disease processes. The solution seemed both simple and profound. Using the principles of five-element acupuncture, I saw cancer as simply an excess of a normal fundamental process. Therefore, the meridian organ system controlling that process must be deficient. My conclusion was to strengthen the deficient system and regain control over the excess. I called this method "the controlling treatment". I believed, at that time, that this was a superior treatment to directly treating the excess, which represents the western medical analogue of suppressing the growth of the tumors (surgery, chemotherapy). I was under the misguided belief that this might hold the key to curing cancer.

In the beginning, the results seemed to prove my theory. In 1984, I first applied a "controlling" treatment method on a dachshund. The dog had multiple tumors along the mammary chain and was struggling to breath, indicative of pulmonary metastasis. Using acupuncture, I treated a strengthening point, LV03, in order to tonify the liver meridian/organ system. As the liver controls the

---

[73] Holistic and spiritual veterinary medicine, Thoresen, Are, 2017. Amazon

stomach meridian (the residence of the mammary chain) such a treatment should take control over the cancer. In a few weeks, the tumors disappeared completely. The dog died several years later from a weakened kidney of old age.

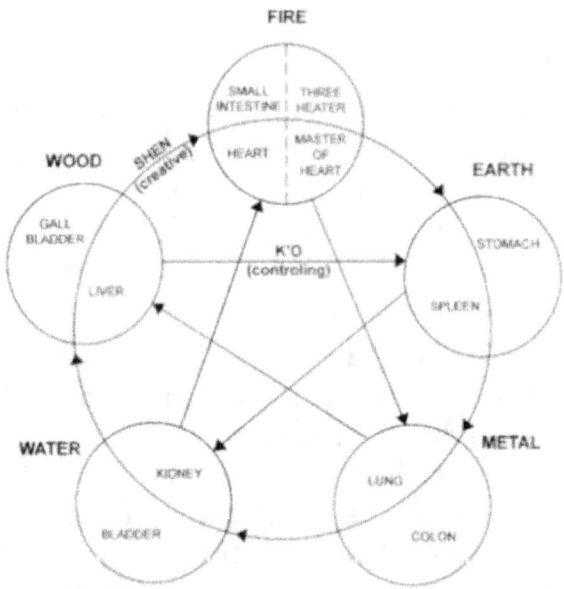

Another example of my success occurred in 1995, when I used this method to treat my first cancer in a horse. My patient was diagnosed with an equine sarcoid, a form of skin cancer. The result was promising, as the sarcoid disappeared within six weeks. With great hope, I published my data in the journal of the Norwegian Veterinary Society.

Since 1984, I have treated more than 1000 patients, suffering from all kinds of cancer, both in animals and humans. The results have been especially good in mammary cancer (85%), and well as in melanoma (80%). Results in lymphosarcoma and brain cancer have been moderately good (70%). However, my results in liver and pancreatic cancer were mediocre; the healing rate being "only" 60% in the few patients I have treated.

My success with treating cancer patients using the controlling method continued for exactly 30 years up until 2014. Then, just after or parallel to my attempts to add the middle-point treatment to my protocols, and also after I visited Israel for the first time, I began to notice a resistance to this particular treatment. Although the tumors would still shrink, the actual ability to cure the patient declined. To make matters even more confusing, my closest students were experiencing the same phenomena. The only group that was still experiencing some success where those physicians that learned the method from my articles rather than directly through me. The efficacy of the controlling method on treating cancer continued to decline throughout 2014 until it was close to non-existent.

I was baffled by this change in events. To create more confusion, the results remained positive when treating other pathologies, unrelated to cancer. In fact, combining the middle point accentuated the positive effect on those patients. I finally realized that it was necessary to re-evaluate the underlying cause of cancer. From the evolution of my studies of Anthroposophic Medicine, I came to the conclusion that all chronic diseases in man are perpetuated by the inhabitancy of Luciferic and Ahrimanic forces. As I have described before, these forces reside in separate regions of the body; the Luciferic entity in the cranial midsection, while the Ahrimanic demon prefers the caudal area. I also discovered that the level of health of the patient was directly correlated to the distance between these two forces. In a relatively healthy state, the distance in a person approximates 20 cm. While in an average horse they are separated by as much as 80 cm. The closer the two entities migrate toward each other, the greater the pathology. Most importantly, I have "seen" that, in cancer, there is a minimal distance between the two, as if they have joined forces. Deductively, I concluded that the effect of these demons is exaggerated by their proximity to one another.

As I started to "see" the disease-bringing demons more often with my spiritual eyes, I understood the importance of translocation in treatment. I realized that most diseases were being treated by addressing one of the two demons: either by weakening or opposing the Luciferic demon (treatment of the excess) or by weakening or opposing the Ahrimanic demon (treatment of the deficiency). I also discovered that both of these methods are more or less symptomatic, often just translocating the pathology to other places in the body or to other humans or animals.

I then developed, as previously described, an understanding of Christ, the Middle-Point and the importance of not fighting the adversaries directly, but transforming them in love, as described in this book. The exact middle-point, where Lucifer and Ahriman join their hands, can be seen in the wooden artwork made by Rudolf Steiner, called "The Group". The hands of the luciferic doppelgänger and the ahrimanic doppelgänger join just below the heart of Christ.

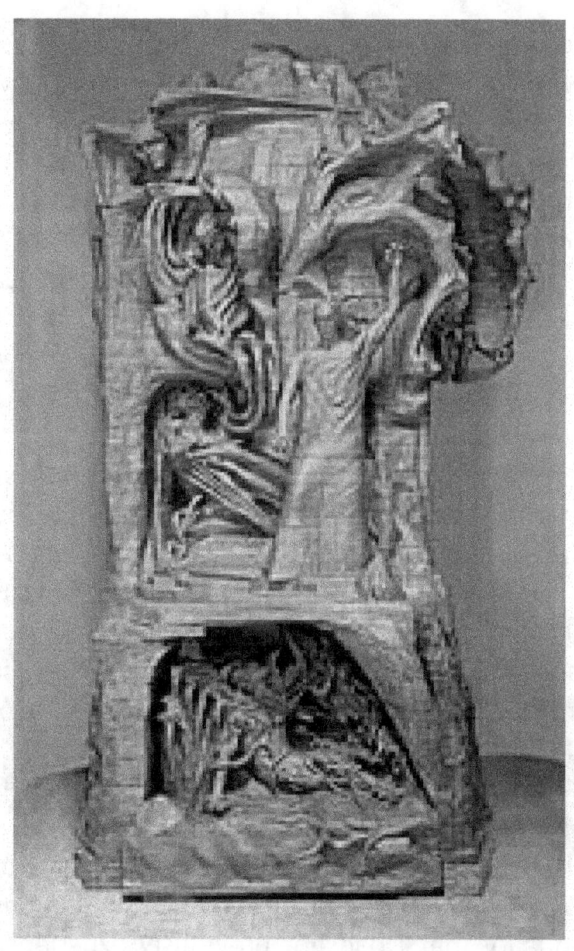

The Group: Christ (representative of man), Lucifer and Ahriman (or their doppelgängers)

Yet, I was left with more questions.

The first question was concerning why these demons were now merging. My personal opinion revolves around my deep belief that the spiritual world is being adversely affected by our material world. Due to "materialism", and the self-centered nature of current humanity at a global level, both Ahrimanic and Luciferic influences are now flourishing.

My second question was regarding why my previous methods stopped working. In regard to this question, I have several theories. I started to entertain the idea that these demons, like any conscious entity, seem to be trying to survive. This natural defensive mechanism lies in direct opposition to their underlying desire to transform into the light. I also realized that to initiate a transformational process, I needed to employ the concept of Christ's love. Finally, I came to the conclusion that when the demons are combined, as in cancer, a different kind of will power was now necessary.

The third question regarded the coincidental emails I began to receive from my students as my results were diminishing. My previous methods stopped working, not only for me, but also for them. I received several from around the world. A Belgium colleague exclaimed that he too, had been experiencing diminishing results regarding cancer treatment. In addition, he relayed a specific story regarding a cat with lymphosarcoma. The more he treated the cat using the appropriate point to treat the deficiency, the more the tumors "translocated" to other meridians. Another example came from a Mexican veterinarian. He explained that when he started using my treatment, his results were excellent but recently, they mysteriously began to fail.

This defensive mechanism displayed by the demons was an emerging quality that I had not previously experienced; which raises the question as to why this was happening. I first assumed that it might lie with me as a healer. Therefore, I theorized that it was a result of either increasing or even decreasing power in my abilities. If it is due to the former, it might be in my ability to use my "spiritual eyes" to visualize such demons and employ the help of Christ consciousness. Therefore, these techniques might have been perceived as a greater threat. If it is due to the latter, it could reside in my past karmic events. Perhaps my atonements for past transgressions was to heal the sick, which was now finally fulfilled. These are only a result of conjecture, as the answer to this question may be forever left unanswered.

A Theoretical Conclusion

In the beginning of 2014 I began to understand the phenomenon of translocation, and how it could be hindered. Because of this newfound knowledge, I changed my protocol of therapy so that the demons were *encouraged* to transform. However, this *encouragement*, met with some resistance. Therefore, I postulated that I needed to use a stronger will to transform the demons that are involved in cancer. It seemed that in other diseases my "loving" encouragement was sufficient.

I now understand that these demons defend themselves. This defensive mechanism could be due to the fact that my resolve in Christ is in opposition to their global survival. Perhaps, it has to do with the ability to "see" them, thus motivating them to try to escape. The third explanation may ultimately have to do with the end of my Karmic debt. Finally, as money is the route of all evil, it may have to do with the greed attached to using the method for profit motive.

My Anthropososophic colleagues also offered some thoughts. A Swedish colleague strongly believed that the increasing cancer rate had to do with a love of money and a lack of spirituality. He believes that cancer itself is a form of healing. A fellow doctor commented on the use of Mistletoe, a remedy used for cancer in Anthroposophic Medicine. He felt that the middle point might be acting like this plant. Steiner saw mistletoe working though Christ consciousness and acting at a spiritual level that may not cure the cancer but allow the patient to "handle it" He also agreed with my theory that my Karma might have been resolved. Finally, a German colleague reminded me that we should always look for the health within the patient and amplify that area. Using Christ's love, we are reminding the patient of the healing that is stored in the body.

Influencing Modalities on Treatment Efficacy

I now understand the importance of a spiritual foundation to my thinking when treating cancer. Spiritual medicine, like quantum physics, is fraught with variability. There are many important factors that can influence the outcome of treatment and influence the resistance of the demons to transform. These are listed below:

1. The geographical location of both the therapist and the patient.
2. The directions of the mountains if they are situated east-west or north-south.
3. The rigidity of the Etheric body of the patient.
4. How much the patient has meditated.
5. The knowledge of the therapist, especially Spiritual knowledge of the Demonic causes of the disease.
6. The karma of both the therapist and the patient.
7. The karma or strength of the disease itself, that is of the Demon(s) causing the disease.
8. The love and empathy between the therapist and the patient.

Examples
1. The personal doctor of Dalai Lama had excellent results with his patients back home in Tibet. However, In Norway, he had limited results, (Himalaya and the Norwegian mountains are not parallel, but oppositely situated.
2. I had no results at all for several years when treating "Herpes Zoster" (Shingles). After reading a lecture of Rudolf Steiner on the spiritual causes and origin of this disease, I had good success for exactly three years, after which, once again, I had no results.

3. When treating cancer with my 5-star control method, I had remarkably better results in treating patients from Switzerland than patients from Norway.
4. I had excellent results in treating breast-cancer in both dogs and humans from 1984 till 2014. Then the results disappeared or changed markedly in the "favor" of the Demons.
5. Rudolf Steiner reported that the effect Dr. Wilhelm Heinrich Schüssler had with his cell salts would last only some years, then the effects would disappear[74].

Despite the unanswered questions, the theories, and the frustration, as you keep reading you will realize that the last words regarding my story of cancer treatment is not yet uttered. The plot thickens with unexpected revelations, when I discover the full strength and meaning of the Middle, Christ and the Group

Later development in acupuncture treatment of cancer

At this point in time, around 2016, I understood clearly that I could not use the five-element cycle as in acupuncture, as there is no Middle Point in the pentagram.

First, I tried with a suggestion from a colleague to make two triangles out of the 'six' processes. This was an interesting suggestion. I have always felt that the combination of both the heart and the pericardium within the Fire process was wrong. I had even tried to modify the five-element star to fit the six yin processes, as six individually divided functions.

---

[74] GA 312, Elfter Vortrag, Dornach, 31. März 1920, page 212.

I divided the heart and the pericardium, and thus created two triangles:

1. HT – KI – LV (the pulses on the left-hand wrist)
2. PC – LU – SP (the pulses on the right-hand wrist)

In these two triangles, the theory was to treat the middle point between the excess and the deficiency pulse.

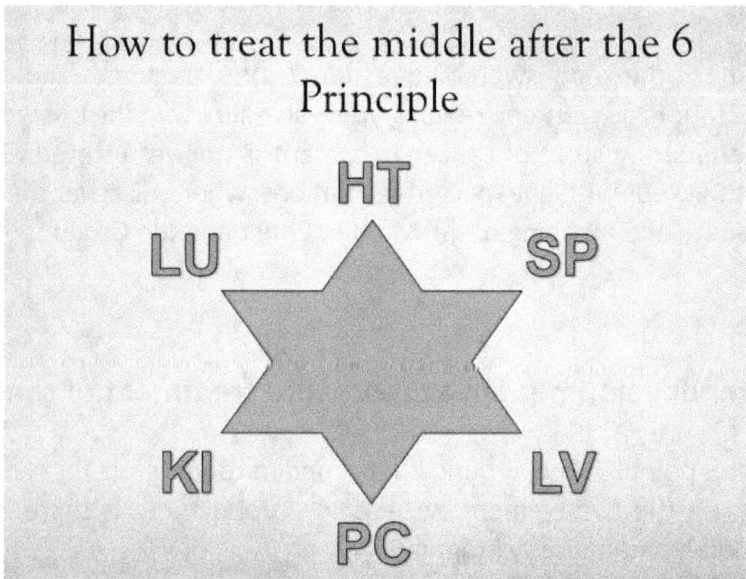

However, I discovered, along with several of my colleagues, that this technique has no therapeutic value.

I understood after a while that I had to rethink Traditional Chinese Medical Theory. I realized that the construction of the 5 elements is designed to treat the excess or deficiency and thereby stimulate further translocation. I concluded that my hypothesis had to be shifted toward an understanding of a post Christian system based on anthroposophy.

According to these principles, the organism teaches us about itself, revealing its characteristics and its interconnectedness with the world that sustains it. This way of doing science enhances our sense of responsibility for nature. As Goethe states, all of nature's individual aspects are interconnected and interdependent. All the parts of an individual have a direct effect on one another, a relationship between one another, thereby constantly renewing the circle of life. Thus, we are justified in considering every animal physiologically perfect. By understanding these tenants, I finally understood that I had to transform the **perceptions** of a pre-Christian system (the law of the five elements) to a post-Christian system, based on anthroposophy. Maybe I could use the Goetheanistic observations of the cosmos and its inhabitants that anthroposophy is so known for?

The most important and fundamental concept in anthroposophy is the 7-fold division of time and of space. I theorized that it would be possible to make two new systems, one based on the 7-foldness of space, and one based on the 7-foldness of time.

Finding the 7-fold system of space (heliocentric and geocentric system).

We relate the spatial relationship of the 7 planets to the 7 organ-meridian processes of Traditional Chinese Medicine. These relationships are recorded in several ancient texts and are shown below;

- Sun: Heart (HT)
- Moon: Reproductive organs (PC)
- Mercury: Intestines, lung (LU, LI, SI)
- Venus: Kidney (KI)
- Mars: Gallbladder (GB)
- Jupiter: Liver (LR or LV)
- Saturn: Spleen (SP)

This represents a total of 7 planets and 7 organ-meridian systems instead of the 5 or 6 organ-meridian systems dealt with by the Chinese. I was then faced with the problem of how to arrange these 7 planets and organs to find the controlling and nourishing sequence as used in the five-element system. After much trial and error, I came down with four possible ways, which I tried to combine in my therapy for two years before I found the 12-element system which now seems to be the most effective, and which also can be combined with the middle point, either individually or in a group.

1. Arrange the 7 elements according to space in the heliocentric system.
2. Arrange the 7 elements according to space in the geocentric system.
3. Arrange the 7 elements according to time in a 7-point star-structure.
4. Arrange the 7 elements according to time in a cradle structure (phasic evolution of the cosmos according to Steiner) I.e.: the downward phase is a mirror of the upward phase.

The Anthroposophic 7 organ-processes in space.

Method 1: The heliocentric system (Processes as the planets are ordered as seen from the sun).

In this system:

- Heart controls Kidney yang (Reproductive organs).
- Kidney yin (the kidney organ itself) controls Liver.
- Gall-bladder controls Heart.
- Lung controls Gall-Bladder.
- Liver controls Lung and Intestines.
- Kidney yang (Reproductive organs) controls Spleen.
- Spleen controls Kidney.

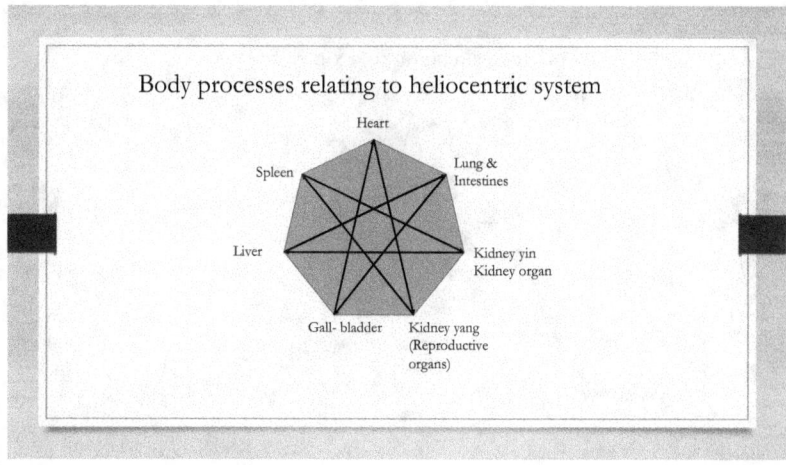

Method 2: The geocentric system (Processes as the planets are ordered as seen from the earth).

In this system:

- Heart controls Spleen.
- Kidney (yin) controls Heart.
- Gall-bladder controls Kidney yin (Kidney).
- Lung (and intestines) controls Gall-bladder.
- Liver controls Lung and intestines.
- Kidney yang (reproductive parts) controls Liver.
- Spleen controls Kidney yang (the adrenals).

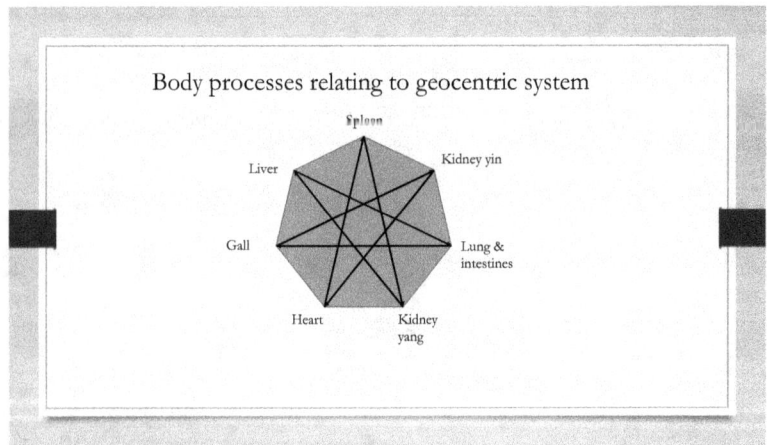

Method 3: Using the order of the planets according to the development of our planetary system, as described by Rudolf Steiner.

In this system:

- Spleen controls Gall-bladder.
- Kidney controls Liver.
- Gall-bladder controls Reproduction (Pericardium).
- Lung controls Spleen.
- Liver controls Heart.
- Pericardium controls Kidney
- Spleen controls Gall-bladder

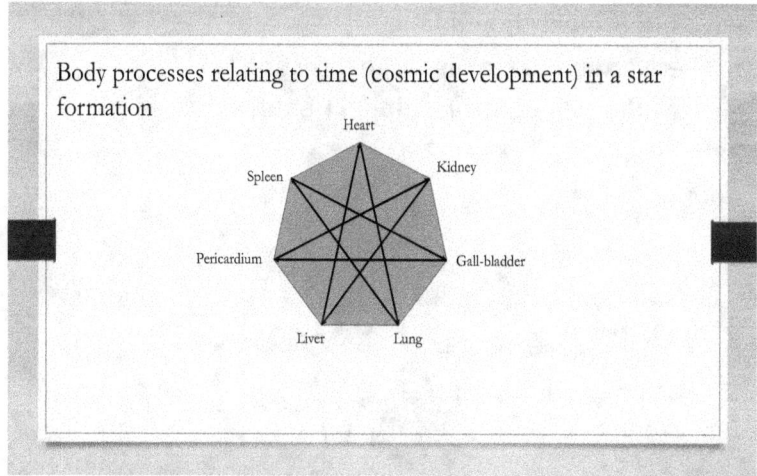

The 12-element zodiacal system.

Method 4: The zodiacal system as viewed as a star (Order of the processes as the zodiacal constellations are arranged in the cosmos).

Where:

- Spleen controls Liver.
- Small Intestine controls Stomach.
- Bladder controls Heart.
- Large Intestine controls Kidney.
- Trippel Heater controls Lung.
- Liver controls Pericardium.
- Stomach controls Gall-bladder.
- Heart controls Spleen.
- Kidney controls Small Intestine.
- Lung controls Bladder.
- Pericardium controls Large Intestine.
- Gall Bladder controls Trippel Heater.

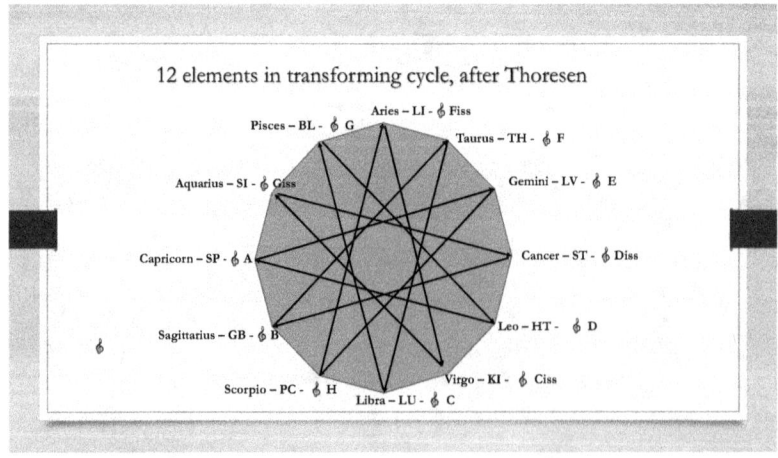

This system I have now used since December 2018, on >1000 patients of all types. The results have been the best I have ever seen, with strong effects and transforming results.

I have not yet had time to make statistics on the effects and results according to the different diseases, but this will be done in the near future.

This system is used like the other systems. If the problem, both the deficiency or the excess, for example is in the liver (LV), then treat this problem with the ting-point of the spleen (SP).[75]

---

[75] Thinking must be used in the initial stage of the diagnosis of any patient, both animal and man. We must inquire about the nature of the disease, make our observations and determine how to perform the treatment. Is surgery needed, is the horse dangerous, can the dog bite us, do we need any medications and so on?

Then we proceed to the method of separating Thinking, Feeling and Willing as described in this book. When we have reached this state of mind, we proceed to focus on the soul faculty of Feeling, visualizing the heart. Here is when we leave the thinking and willing behind. We imagine spiritually entering the 12th layer of the heart of the patient. We imagine a tunnel from our heart to the heart of the patient. This tunnel traverses all 12 layers of the body coming to an end at the center of the patient's heart.

Keeping our focus here, we make our diagnosis. Personally, I use the pulse-diagnosis to go through all the different processes of the body, both in the present time and in the past, however any modality of Spiritual diagnosis may be used whether it be homeopathy, kinesiology or any method that may give the information we need. We can also go into the processes of the forefathers and foremothers, investigating the different physical, mental or spiritual traumas. In doing this, we mentally organize the information that we have gathered. This is when we combine the Thinking with the Feeling.

When we have decided with our Thinking how to treat the disease, we leave both the thinking and the feeling behind, and enter into the Will power of the universe, which is to be found in the earth itself. This Will force must be used in the therapeutic part of the procedure. The focus of the therapist will then be in his limbs, his feet, or even in the earth beneath his feet. From this area, the force of the Will is awakened, and this force will then stream up through the body. The path this force takes is not along the spine, described as the "Kundalini" force in old traditions. This up-going stream should be found in

The appearance of the 3 double-crosses in the 12-element controlling circle. A possible transition from pre- to post-Christian thinking.

If we look carefully on the structure of the 12-star, we will soon realize an interesting geometric pattern. The structure actually consists of 3 crosses, each formed as a double-cross.

The first cross consists of the axis of the BL to LI and LU to KI, crossed with the horizontal axis of SP to GB and LV to ST. All the diagonals in this cross are acupuncture Yin-Yang pairs.

The second cross consists of the axis of the SI to the BL and the KI to the HT, crossed with the horizontal axis of GB to PC and TH to LV. All the diagonals in this cross are within acupuncture Yin-Yang pairs.

---

front of the spine. The force in the spine is of the old world, related to Lucifer. The force of the new world is in the middle of the body, related to Christ. It is possible to experience this up-going stream as a dance between two snakes, one white and one black. This force must then enter the heart and mingle with the feeling, compassion and love for the patient, and, in fact, for the whole of humanity. If we activate the Kundalini force, this goes straight to the crown chakra, and does not stop at the level of the heart. This mingling often results in a feeling of Cosmic divine love, inhabiting the center of the heart. From this center, the healing force, now totally cleaned from any egoistic wish or intent, streams over into the patient. Here, directed by intentional thought that streams down from the head, the healing force works in the body by diminishing the power of the Demons. If this force is directed against the ahrimanic demon, the healing of the organic structures will begin. If it is directed against the luciferic demon, the pain and unpleasantness will diminish. If it is directed to the Middle, the Christ-Point or the Christ-filled gap between the two Demons, both Demons will pull back and start to dissolve or Transform.

The third cross consists of the axis SP-SI and HT-ST, crossed with the horizontal axis of PC-LU and LI-TH. All the diagonals in this third cross are again within acupuncture Yin-Yang pairs.

The KVINT-circle and the countercurrent CROMATIC circle that appear in the 12-element zodiacal transformative circle.

I have for many years studied the relationship between the 12 tones in our scale and the zodiacal constellations.

Likewise, I have also studied the relationship between the acupuncture meridians and the musical tones.

- There are 12 meridians
- There are 12 zodiacal signs
- There are 12 tones in our music

When we have arranged in a circle as showed above, the zodiacal signs as a continuous succession, just as in the cosmos, we get the succession as follows, starting with Libra: Libra - Scorpio - Sagittarius - Capricorn - Aquarius - Pisces - Aries - Taurus - Gemini - Cancer - Leo - Virgo.

If we then add the relating meridians to this succession we get the following line: LU - PC - GB - SP - SI - BL - LI - TH - LV - ST - HT - KI.

We also see from the figure of the 12 signs that the controlling functions (the lines in the star-formation) are related to the KVINT, as the succession of musical tones are as follows: C - H - B - A - Giss - G - Fiss - F - E - Diss - D - Ciss.

For example, we see that as LU is controlling BL, then the related tones will be C and G, which constitutes a KVINT. And so it is with all the meridians and tones.

Also, it is worthwhile to observe that if we follow the notes counterclockwise, we get the CROMATIC scale of C - Ciss - D - Diss - E - F - Fiss - G - Giss - A - B - H and again C.

The appearance of the 3 single-crosses in the 12-element controlling circle. A possible description of the power-flow of the universe.

If we look carefully at the structure of the 12-star, we will soon begin to realize an even more interesting geometric pattern. The structure actually consists of 3 single crosses, each expressing the power-constellations of the cosmos.

1. The first cross consists of the axis of the BL to KI, crossed with the horizontal axis of LV to GB. This cross relates, according to Rudolf Steiner, to the morning – evening – axis of Christ (Pisces) and Sophia (Virgo), which are positive forces. This axis is then crossed by the diagonal of midday – midnight, of Ahriman (Gemini) and Lucifer (Sagittarius), which are evil forces.
2. The second cross consisting of the axis of the LI to LU, being crossed by SP to ST.
3. The third cross consists of the axis of the TH to PC, being crossed by SI to HT.

These relations offer us another insight into a controlling and transforming therapy, which will be explained after the following quotation of Rudolf Steiner.

If we take a closer look at the **spiritual forces** emanating from the different constellations, we find Steiners words[76] somewhat enlightening:

> *And so, just as it is essential for an orthodox professor of biology to have the most powerful microscope available and the most efficient laboratory methods, so, in the future, when science has been spiritualized, it will be of the utmost importance whether certain processes are carried through in the morning or in the evening, or at midday, and whether what has been done in the morning is allowed to be further influenced by an evening activity, or whether the cosmic influences are cut out, paralyzed, from the morning until the evening. Processes of this kind will of necessity come to light and will run their course. Naturally, a great deal of water will have to flow under the bridges before the professional chairs and laboratories, at present organized on purely materialistic lines, are handed over to spiritual scientists, but this replacement must come about if humanity is not to sink into utter decadence. For example, if the question is one of doing good in the immediate future, existing laboratory methods must give way to methods whereby certain processes take place in the morning and are interrupted during the day, so that the cosmic stream passes through them again in the evening and is in turn rhythmically withheld again until morning. So, the processes would take their course: certain cosmic workings would always be interrupted by day, and the cosmic morning and evening processes would be brought in. All sorts of arrangements would be necessary for this.*

---

[76] «Reappearance of Christ in the Etheric", lecture 12, held on the 25th of November 1917, by Rudolf Steiner, GA 178.

You will realize that if one is not in a position to take any public action about these things, all one can do is to speak of them.

However, just as gold, health and the prolongation of life are put in the place of God, virtue and immortality, so from the same quarter efforts will be made to work not with the morning and evening processes, but with others. Last week I told you how an attempt will be made to set aside the impulse of the Mystery of Golgotha, while for the West another impulse, a sort of Antichrist is introduced; and from the East an attempt will be made to paralyze the twentieth century manifestation of the Christ Impulse by diverting attention from the coming etheric Christ.

Those concerned to present an Anti-Christ as the real Christ will try also to make use of something that works through the most material forces, but in this very way can work spiritually. Above all they will strive to make use of electricity and earth-magnetism in order to produce effects all over the world. I have shown you how earth-forces rise up into what I have called the human Double, the Doppelgänger. This secret will be opened up. An American secret will be to make use of earth-magnetism, with its north-south duality, and by this means to send over the earth guiding forces which will have spiritual effects. Look at the magnetic chart of the earth and compare it with what I am now saying. Observe where the magnetic needle deviates to East and West and where it does not deviate. I can give only hints about all this. From a certain direction in the heavens, spiritual beings are continually active, and they have only to be put into the service of the earth, and — because these beings working in from the cosmos can mediate the secret of the earth's magnetism — it will be possible for egotistic groups to get behind this secret and to accomplish a great deal in connection with gold, health and the prolongation of life. It will be necessary for them only to pluck up their faltering courage — and in certain circles that will be done readily enough!

From the East an endeavor will be made to strengthen what I have already explained: to place in the service of the earth the beings which work in from the opposite side of the cosmos. In the future there will be a great battle. Human science will stretch out to the cosmic, but will try to get there by different paths. It will be the task of good, healing science to find certain cosmic forces which can reach the earth through the co-operation of two cosmic streams, those of Pisces and Virgo. The great secret to be discovered will be how the influence which works from the direction of Pisces as a power of the sun unites itself with the influence working from the direction of Virgo. It will make for good when it is learnt how the morning and evening forces from the two sides of the cosmos can be brought into the service of humanity.

These forces, however, will be left aside by those who try to achieve their whole purpose through the polaric duality of positive and negative forces. The forces which enable the spiritual to stream down to earth with the aid of positive and negative magnetism come from Gemini; they are the midday forces. In ancient times it was known that cosmic influences were involved in this, and to-day even exoteric scientists are aware that in some or other way positive and negative magnetism lie behind Gemini in the Zodiac. The aim will be to paralyze all that could be gained through a revelation of the true duality in the cosmos — to paralyze it in a materialistic, egotistic way by means of the forces which stream in particularly from Gemini and can be placed entirely at the service of the human "Double."

Other brotherhoods, concerned above all to divert attention from the Mystery of Golgotha, will try to make use of the duality in human nature — the duality which in our epoch embraces man as a unity, but includes within him his lower animal nature. A human being is really a centaur in a certain sense: his humanity rests on his lower animal nature in its astral form. This working together of the duality in man gives rise to a duality of forces. This duality of forces will be utilized particularly by certain egotistic brotherhoods, chiefly from the side of India and the East, in order to mislead eastern Europe, whose task it is to prepare for the sixth post-Atlantean epoch. And this will be done with the aid of the forces which work in from Sagittarius.

Be aware of the three single crosses.

Our 'logical' conception of reality in making everything into polarities is for me like being dragged into Maya, as I consider the middle to be the only force of reality, our only salvation.

The polarities seem to me to be an expression of the great illusion, whilst the trinity expresses the reality.

It is of vital importance to find this third aspect in all uses of electricity, magnetism, nuclear power, cosmic streams or corporeal balances, otherwise the ahrimanic-luciferic forces will dominate.

We find the same opposition between duality and trinity in the soul forces of thinking, feeling and willing. Within each we must find the middle point, the middle force, and if we can then relate to and use this middle, this force of LOVE as a fourth force permeating the cosmos, we have a cross, similar to the morning-evening-midday-midnight forces.

The only salvation is to add the force of LOVE to the fundamental forces.

That is why the symbol reflecting the love of Jesus Christ is a CROSS.

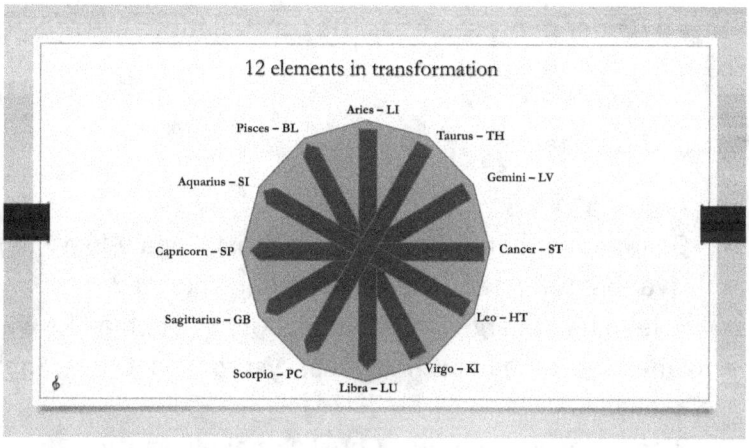

How the middle can heal the adversarial forces.

Here we see a picture of the main opposing forces represented by the line between Pisces and Virgo and the opposing or adversary forces exposing themselves in the line between Sagittarius and Gemini.

The interesting observation is that the healing forces from Pisces (Christ) can transform the forces of Gemini (Ahriman), and the healing forces of Virgo (Sophia) can heal the adversarial forces of

Sagittarius (Lucifer), and that these healing forces arrive in a 90^0 (degree) angel.

The next two pages illustrate how this healing force can be extended to cover all the different constellations, bearing in mind that the healing forces always arrive in a 90^0 (degree) angel.

Here we see how this healing force can be active through the whole circle of organs or stellar forces.

The 12-element zodiacal system.

Method 5: The zodiacal system as viewed as a quadratum (in a 90^0 angel) (Order of processes as the constellations are ordered in the cosmos).

Where in this system:

- Gall-bladder heals Bladder (in a Christ/Sophia-like way).
- Liver heals Kidney (in a Christ/Sophia-like way).
- Spleen heals Large Intestine (in a Christ/Sophia-like way).
- Small Intestine heals hormonal system (in a Christ/Sophia-like way).
- Bladder heals Liver (in a Christ/Sophia-like way).
- Large Intestine heals Stomach (in a Christ/Sophia-like way).
- hormonal system heals Heart (in a Christ/Sophia-like way).
- Liver heals Kidney (in a Christ/Sophia-like way).
- Stomach heals Lung (in a Christ/Sophia-like way).
- Heart heals Pericardium (in a Christ/Sophia-like way).
- Kidney heals Gall bladder (in a Christ/Sophia-like way).
- Lung heals Spleen (in a Christ/Sophia-like way).

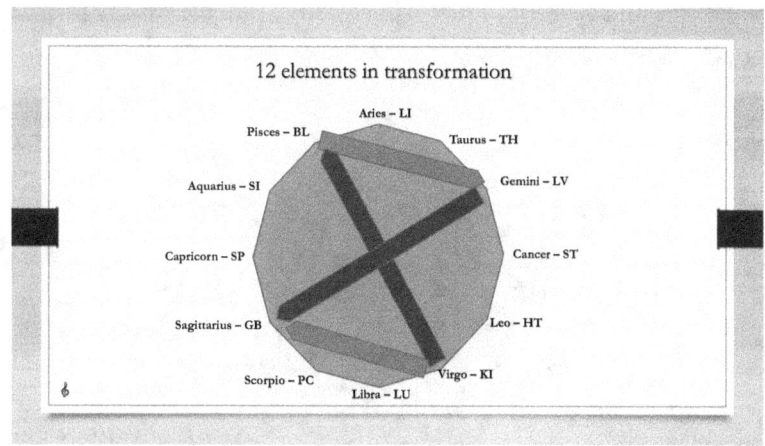

In this system we have 3 quadrats:

4. Hormonal system – Heart – Pericardium – Small Intestine.
    This is the feeling-inter(by love)-healing-system.
5. Liver – Kidney – Gall bladder – Bladder.
    This is the willing-inter(by love)-healing-system.
6. Stomach – Lung – Spleen – Large intestine.
    This is the thinking-inter(by love)-healing-system.

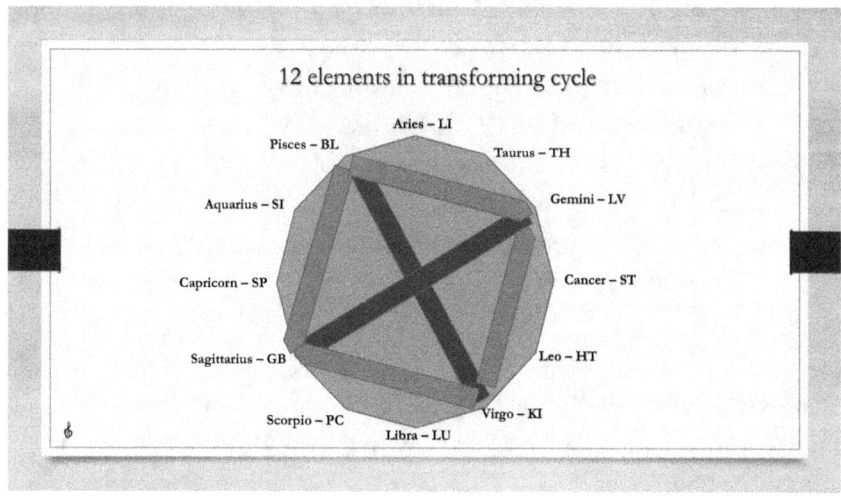

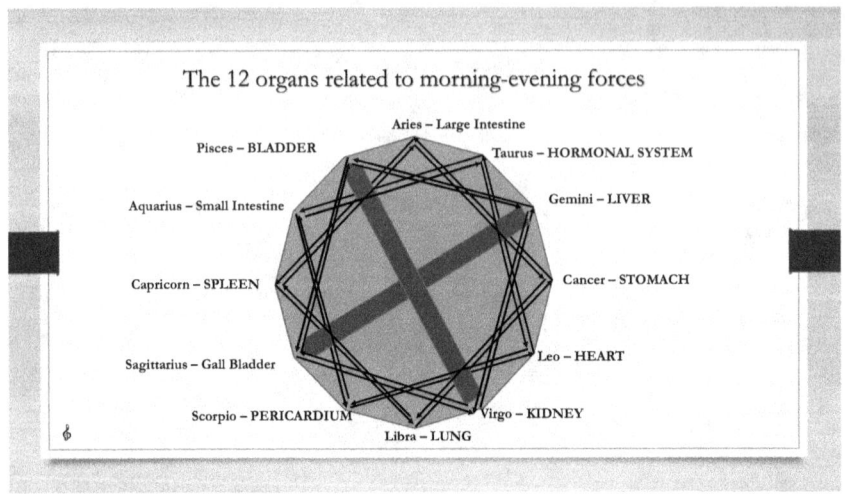

Where in this system:

- Liver and Gall-bladder heals Kidney and Bladder (in a Christ/Sophia-like way).
- Kidney and Bladder heals Liver and gall-bladder (in a Christ/Sophia-like way).
- Heart and Small Intestine heals Pericardium and Trippel Heather (in a Christ/Sophia-like way).
- Pericardium and Trippel Heather heals Heart and Small Intestine (in a Christ/Sophia-like way).
- Lung and Large Intestine heals Spleen and Stomach (in a Christ/Sophia-like way).
- Spleen and Stomach heals Lung and Large Intestine (in a Christ/Sophia-like way).

An explanation to the last figure.
Here, in this last figure we see how the masculine and feminine forces together can heal.
First, we had separated the masculine and the feminine from the 5-elemets to a 12 element-cycle, where the masculine and the feminine had been separated, and then, as shown in the last figure,

both the masculine and the feminine can work together in healing the disease.

In this way liver and gall bladder can together heal both the kidney and the bladder.

In this way we will have:
4. Liver and Gallbladder together heals Kidney and Bladder and vica versa.
5. Lung and large Intestine together heals Spleen and Stomach and vica versa.
6. Heart and Small intestine together heals pericardium and Hormonal system and vica versa.

In this way man and woman, Christ and Sophia, join their forces in healing the world.

Salvatore Mundi.

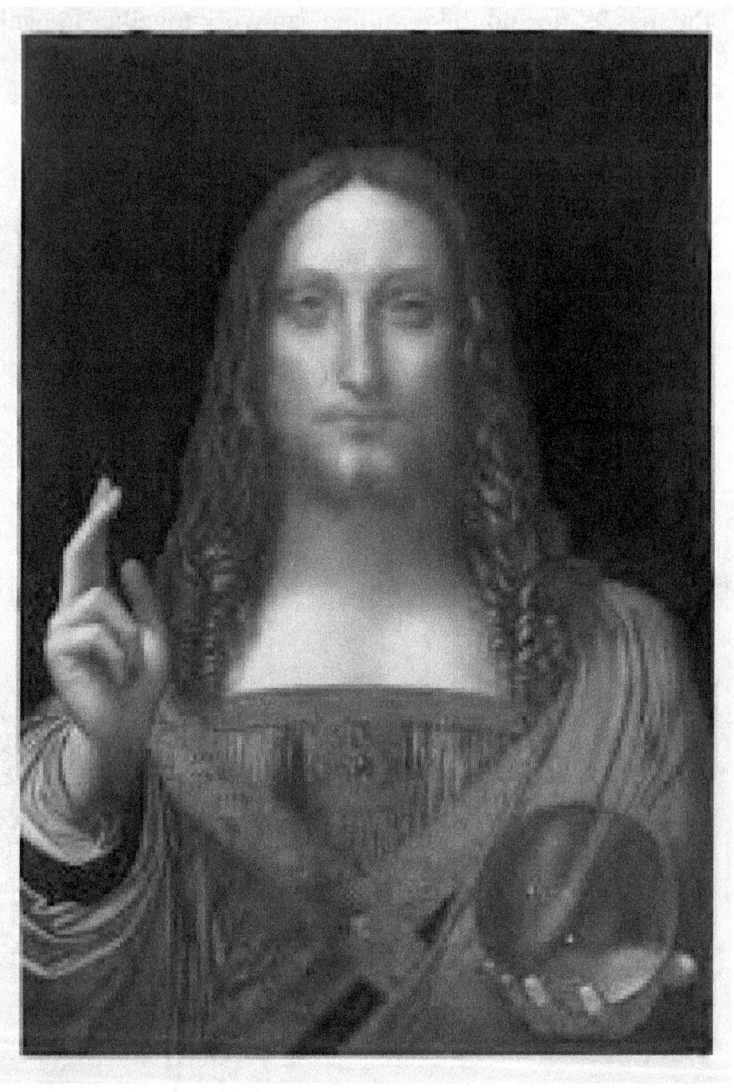

Chapter 18:

More about the middle and Finding the Middle Point

1. Seeing the middle point:(Clairvoyance)

The ability to "see" the spiritual world can be a natural gift or, with dedication, it can be learned. For me, it was a skill that I possessed since I was born. In my early youth, it felt so natural, that I assumed that everyone had this ability.

Although I use the word "see", this does not exactly convey the experience, as the physical eyes are not involved. For lack of a better description, this is as close a word I can use to describe the phenomenon. In order to gain access to the spiritual world, it is necessary to be able to excarnate from the material body. For me, this was a state that would happen quite frequently without conscious effort. After studying Anthroposophy, I discovered this was the product of a separation of feeling, thinking and willing. According to Rudolf Steiner, this is the method that allows one, that is not naturally gifted with such a talent, to learn to spiritually "see". Later in life I learned to create these excarnations using the techniques I have earlier described. With my spiritual eyes, I am then able to perceive the presence and location of these Ahrimanic and Luciferic structures and find the point residing midpoint between their locations.

According to Rudolf Steiner there is another divisional hierarchy that can be separated to obtain the state of clairvoyance. Steiner uses the term body in a broader sense than the typical definition. He uses it to describe the human existence that represents a single lifetime. The first most obvious division within the body of man is the actual human material body. The next layer involves that which permeates our physicality with the forces of life that regulate and maintain the development of the physical form. This is referred to as the etheric body, found in all living things including plants. The third subtle body is the astral, which represents the emotions and feelings of a consciousness that is present in only man and animal. Finally, there is the division of the ego or I consciousness, which represents the faculty of self-awareness, a trait unique to man. The three subtle bodies of etheric, astral, and I consciousness separate during sleep. The latter two, are the framework for our soul experience, but during the sleep state, they are suppressed. Therefore, one is unable to experience the external world necessary for any form of development. However, If we could reproduce a condition which resembles sleep, yet remain conscious of our surroundings, we might be able to reach super sensible knowledge. This would be similar to a daydream where a vivid inner life would be allowed to unfold. This is the condition that can allow clairvoyance.

The easiest of the above two methods is the separation of feeling, thinking and willing. As discussed thoroughly in Chapter 1, these three divine forces actually do not originate from our body, but from the spirit world. As we incarnate, these faculties are intermingled and bound together and are therefore hidden from us. In order to develop our spiritual eye, we must learn to separate them through understanding their origin, as well as the performance of specific exercises and meditations[77]

2. Feeling the middle point (clairsentience).

This is the ability to receive information through sensing or feeling subtle energy. It is actually one of the more common psychic gifts often activated without conscious awareness. Loosely translated it means a "clear feeling". Clairsentience can trigger physical sensations such as tingling, a ringing in the ear, or changes in the

---

[77] The knowledge of the true origin of Thinking, Feeling and Willing are described by many mystics and in many of the mysteries through the ages, among others by Rudolf Steiner in his Anthroposophy.

practitioner's pulse. In extreme cases, one can even feel physical pain.

For some students, using Nogiér's pulse diagnosis to find the middle point is a form of effective clairsentience[78]. Nogiér, A French acupuncturist known for the development of auricular acupuncture, used the pulse as a kind of "Geiger counter" to find various pathologies. When a honing device was passed over a testing zone, the practitioners pulse, taken at the auricular artery would change in rate or intensity. Using this same concept, one can pass the finger of one hand over the mid-section, while taking the auricular pulse with the other hand, and wait for a change in intensity or frequency.

Others have found that while performing this procedure, the patient often exhibits or experiences a change when the practitioner's finger is passed across the middle point. Horses are particularly sensitive and can be observed to chew, drop their heads and/or blink and close their eyes.

For many practitioners, the simple act of feeling the area can be informative. Some feel changes in temperature, while others feel a kind of roughness to the skin that, at a physical level, may not be overtly palpable.

3. Smelling the Middle Point:(Clairalience[79])

During the winter of 2017 I was teaching courses on how to find and treat the middle in both New York and Florida. In New York I had a student who claimed to have the ability to smell the

---

[78] Auriculotherapy manual Chinese and western systems of ear acupuncture, Oleson, Terry, 2014, google books.

[79] Clairalience: (Clair meaning "Clear" and "Alience" meaning scent) is the Psychic ability to be able to obtain specific Psychic information based on your use of the scent of smell. It along with its sister abilities (Clairaudience, Clairvoyance, Claircognizance and Clairsentience) make up 5 of the 6 Psychic sense abilities.

presence of disease. With that proclamation, she insisted on smelling each patient to find the middle point. As I then proceeded to Florida to teach yet another group, I discovered that most did not possess the ability to spiritually see the middle point. It was at this point that I decided to test the efficacy of Clairalience. I began by emptying my lungs of air and then with one long inhalation I passed my nostrils along the midsection of a canine patient. Much to my surprise, I found a clear change in the odour at the level of the midpoint. At the exact location, the odour changed from a normal dog smell to a more pleasant aroma. Continuing beyond the point, however, revealed a pathological smell, quite distinct from the middle scent. After interviewing the course participants, I found that some were able to distinguish these three odors. I coined the phrase "the sniffing diagnostic test" for my new method of finding the middle point

The exact method involves exhaling all the air from the lung, and with a long and constant inhalation through the nose move the head in a steady pace, over the back of the patient as shown below. To my surprise, I found it to be quite simple for me and several of the students to smell the middle point. Cranial to the Middle Point the smell is very typical. At the exact Middle Point, the smell changed to a pleasant odor, and immediately caudal to the Middle, the smell again changed to a somewhat more "physical", dog like, or even pathological smell. I asked the other participants to do this "sniffing-test", and about 30% of the participants could clearly recognize the 3 different smells.

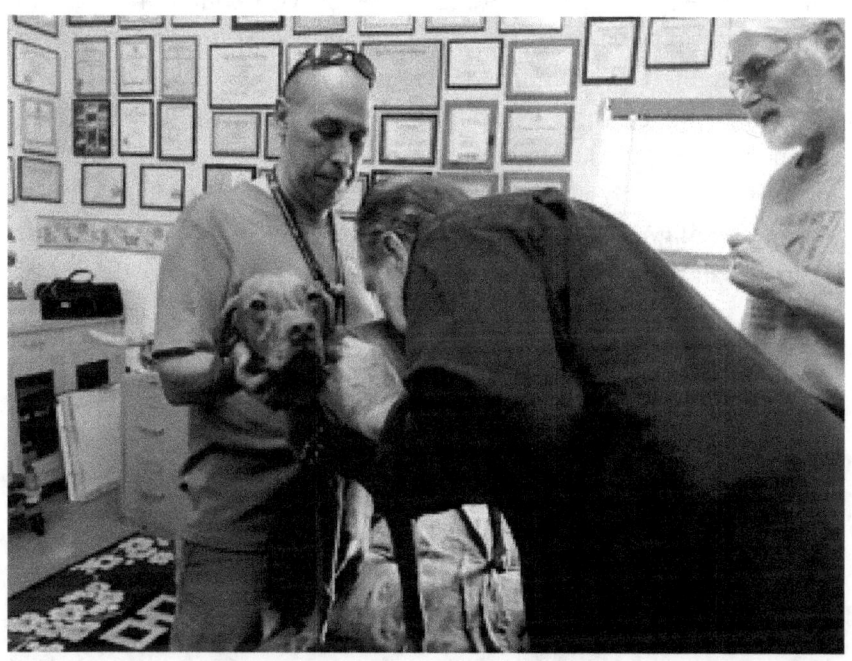

the "sniffing diagnostic test".

Using the Middle point to treat noxious earth radiation

Earth-Radiation appears to my Spiritual eye, as black snakes curling and moving along the surface of the earth. They must not be mistaken for the energetic bonds between trees and plants, which are described in my book "Poplar". These bonds, although similar in their movement along the forest floor, are much lighter in hue.

I have been able to enter these "tree snakes" with my consciousness, and as such, can travel within this energy pattern. Travelling in the left direction takes me back in time. I have never attempted to Travel to the right for fear of seeing the future. I consider the future belonging to higher powers than mine. Within the energetic streams of the trees, I have experienced the secret of the "double time stream".[80]

The black snakes that are the expression of Earth-Radiation are 'seen' as darker and not as transparent as the tree energy snakes. Entering inside the earth-radiation snakes is not advisable, as they are of a malignant Ahrimanic nature. They represent the past deeds of all humans, the karma of each of each and every one of us. This karma of past deeds can be healed by asking forgiveness in the name of Christ.

Using the Middle Point to treat plants and trees

For many years I have been able to "pulse" trees. A German colleague, Ferdinand Niessen, told me he felt that all trees had a weakness in the water element about one third distal to the top of its structure. I pondered this phenomenon for years until I realized that all humans and animals have a deficiency of water where Lucifer abides, which is the top half of the body. As Lucifer represents heat, we often find a deficient kidney energy in that area.

One third proximal to the root of the tree, and one third cranial to the tail base of animals and humans, we can find the Ahrimanic influence. Here there is a deficiency in the wood element, representing the energy and fundamental process of the liver as defined by Five Element Acupuncture.

Therefore, when we pulse a tree, it is important that we do not pulse the tree 1/3 from the root or 1/3 from the top, otherwise we always get either a deficiency in the liver or in the kidney. In animals and humans this is the same. We have to focus and

---

[80] **The double time stream** is one of the most important secrets we have to know about when entering the Spiritual world. Time can go either way, both from the future towards the past, and from the past against the future.

spiritually enter the heart of the patient to get a correct pulse finding.

To treat a tree from the Middle-Point, we "needle it mentally" on the Middle Point between the kidney-deficiency and the liver-deficiency. When I do this, I find that both the deficiencies often disappear.

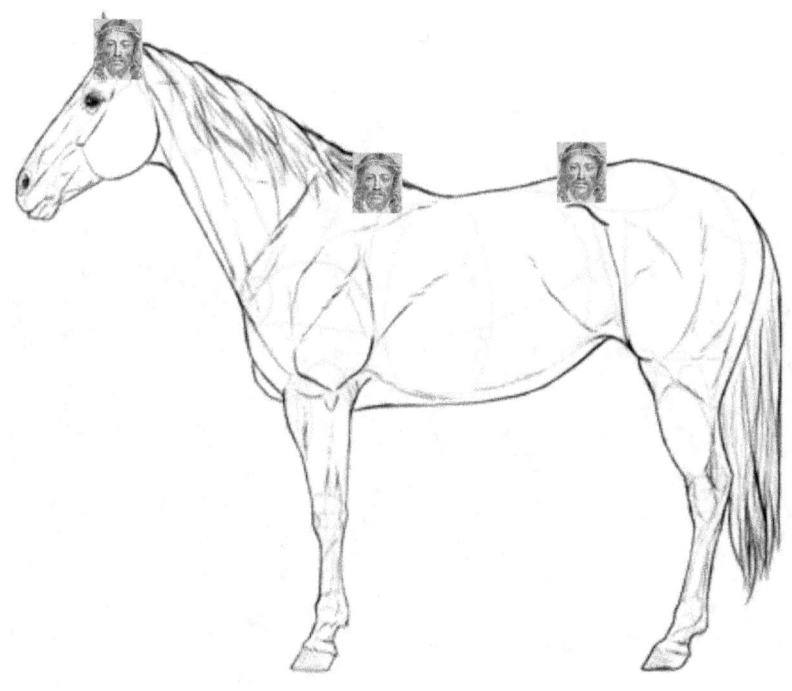

Chapter 19:

The Importance of the Group

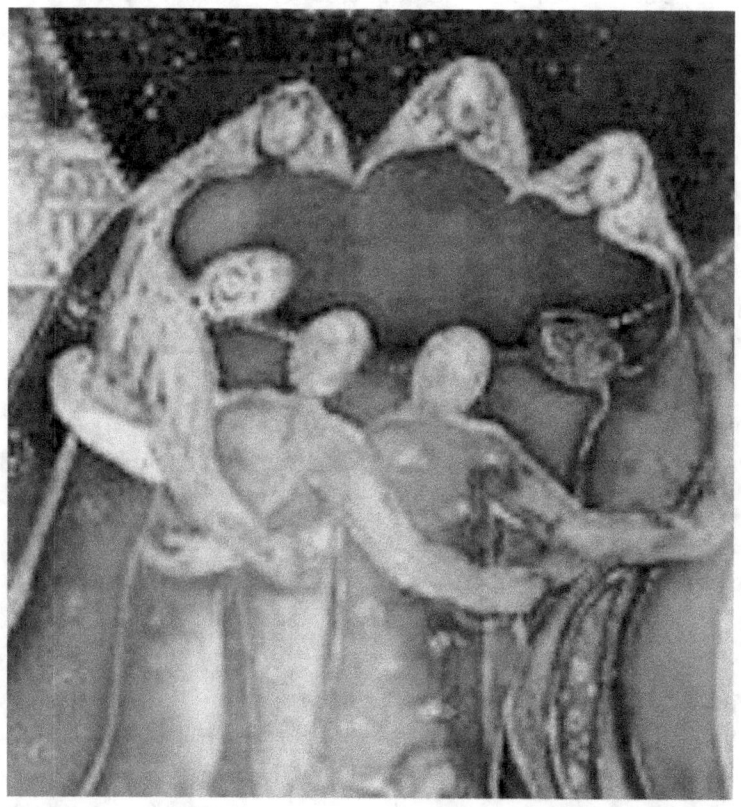

On the evening of November 5th, 2016, something unexpected happened. I was giving a veterinary course in New York and decided to treat the participants with the middle point. Twenty-five participants were lying on the floor as I needled all the individual midpoints between Lucifer and Ahriman. Then I sat back to watch. The needle that was placed on the thorax, between the adversaries, seemed to activate the area of "free" etheric force, not dominated by Ahriman or Lucifer. This area became activated as a light that emanated from it was rhythmically oscillating. After some time, the demons also became light-filled and started to float up from the participants to circle around and over the entire group. The circling became more and more luminous going upwards in a stream. In the light, the face of an Angel appeared. One of the participants visualized the archangel Michael. I went into the middle of the whirling light and felt divine.

The needling of the Middle point apparently caused an oscillation in the etheric bodies of the participants just between the Ahrimanic and the Luciferic pathological structures. This oscillation in the different patients started to create a sympathetic resonance among the members of the group, and this resonance multiplied the strength of the treatment to a very high degree, so that the whole group was drawn into the effect of the treatment, even those where the Ahrimanic and the Luciferic Demons were tightly bound together, as they are in cancer. What I could not have done in such patients, was done through the whole group.

What I saw happening with the group was totally different from what happens when I treat an individual. I suddenly realized what was happening to the group, as if I was struck by a heavenly light. The additional strength of conjoined demons could not withstand the power of the combined activated energy of the group. The cooperation of the good in each and every one of the patients was able to transform evil into light.

I also discovered modalities relating to the effect that I visualized. It is stronger at dawn and dusk, and having the patients lie in an east-west direction. These attributes are a part of the attributes of etheric energy in general. I have always had a better result in treating cancer in patients coming from areas of the world where the mountains were directed east-west (Alps, Himalaya) than from those coming from areas where the mountains are directed north-south (Norway, USA).

The Fallacy of Individualization

The irony of individualized treatment then became apparent. It was obvious that Ahrimanic forces are enhanced when man is "culled from the group". Sadly, the individualized approach to cancer treatment has become the gold standard, especially with regards to immunotherapy. Without an understanding of spiritual science, the medical community is unaware of the power they are giving to the adversarial forces that perpetuate this disease.

This strategy to divide and conquer is used by more sinister occult groups who employ black magic to steal etheric energy from single individuals through different kinds of treatments, procedures or rituals. I have met with two such groups: the Thule-group in Germany and the Damanhur-group in Italy.

Several years ago, I accepted an invitation to visit a professor of a German organization called The Thule-group. They were organizing and operating a large alternative healing school in Scandinavia. On the first day of the visit I came to the frightening realization that most of the patients at his clinic were Nazis of various ages. But the most terrifying incident occurred on the last day of the visit, when the professor I was visiting invited me to a private dinner at his house. As I entered his home I was immediately faced with a huge painting of Christ on the cross, hanging with his feet up. If that wasn't disconcerting enough, during the dinner I saw, with my spiritual eyes, a small wall photograph pulsating negative energy towards the professor. When I told him what was happening, he got up from the table and turned the picture to hide the photograph that was being displayed. Quite to my surprise, the professor immediately fell onto the floor. I came to his aide and resuscitated him. After he recovered, he was so convinced that I had saved his life, that he confided in me and told me the true story of the Thule-group. He revealed that the organization practiced black magic. For every healing their students did, a certain part of the patient's energy was used by the leaders of this group for their own dark purposes.

In hindsight, I now realize this was a perfect example of demon translocation in an individual.

Many years later, The Damanhur-group came to Norway to build special stone labyrinths. They were quite forth telling on the intended purpose of the stones they were crafting. Any one entering the labyrinths would have their energy siphoned to be transferred to the "Selfic" temple-room in Northern Italy. They even admitted that this energy was to be used by their leaders for the purposes of their choosing. This is one of the many ways that the adversaries try to gain control over the etheric forces and powers in their fight against all that is good.

The Fallacy of Mechanization

Rudolf Steiner, the father of Anthroposophy, predicted in the beginning of the 20th century, that mankind will become increasingly infused with technology. He also believed that this technology would be utilized by the adversaries to gain access and control over all of human evolution. He was correct. Mechanization is another means by which ahrimanic forces can fortify their hold on the material world.

Once again, it cannot be under stated that by using the social element of a group treatment, combined with the absence of machines; and by using only one single needle in the healthiest point of the body, namely the Christ point; we can go forward in preventing the disastrous cooperation between Lucifer and Ahriman. In this way, we can prevent the epidemic wave of cancer we see today. Hopefully, as the medical community sees the importance of Spiritual Science in healing, we can then begin to cure all who suffer on this planet.

The Group wooden sculpture of Rudolf Steiner.

Housed in the Gotheanum, in Dornach, Switzerland, lives the Group. Born from the imagination of Rudolf Steiner and a sculptor named Edith Maryon, this is a wooden sculpture of Christ as the representative of humanity, standing in between Lucifer and Ahriman with arms outstretched as if keeping them apart and controlled. This enormous work of art, elegantly sums up the plight and redemption of mankind.

As I explained earlier, studying this sculpture gave me many of my insights regarding treating with the Christ point. As can be seen in the following pictures, the exact middle point, where Lucifer and Ahriman join their hands, lies just below the level of the heart of Christ. However, in this sculpture, there are several more secrets to be found. These are secrets that may reveal, strengthen and make clear the therapeutic possibilities that we can utilize to combat and transform these demons. These are some of my insights obtained from studying this statue:

1. Christ is the dividing force between Lucifer and Ahriman.
2. the cooperation or combination of these two forces poses a sincere threat to human kind.
3. The Luciferic and the Ahrimanic forces join below the heart of Christ (and for that matter, man).
4. There are two Ahrimans and two Lucifers, so that the meeting points between them in the body are in two places, one under the heart and one at the level of the throat.
5. The "Cosmic Humour" appears when there is a group gathered, in celebration of the Christ healing force.

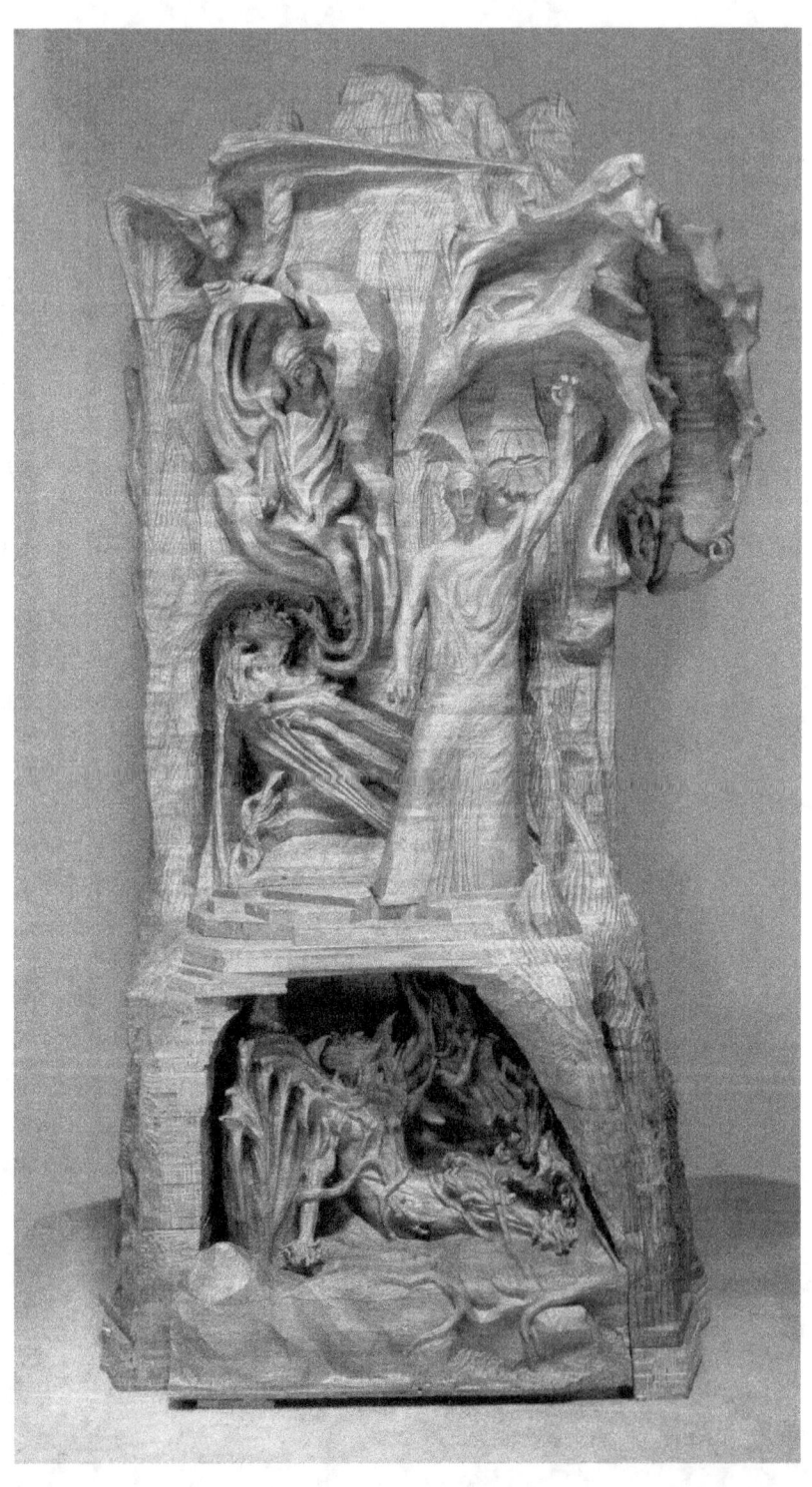

Chapter 20:

Classical Homeopathy in Anthroposophic Medicine by Margaret Mary Fleming, D.V.M, A.P.

To understand homeopathy is to understand its roots. At the beginning of the 19th century, a German physician named Samuel Hahnemann, otherwise known as the father of homeopathy, spent his entire adult life as a medical physician, horrified by the tortuous methods of treatment in his day. As a result, he began a search for an effective alternative that would not only alleviate suffering but do so using easily understandable and fundamental principles as described below.

He dubbed this form of healing "homeopathy" a Greek phrase meaning "similar suffering". Hahnemann presented the essence of his curative system as a complete therapeutic method of the treatment of disease, and in his crowning achievement, he wrote a book he entitled "the Organon[81]". Here, he painstakingly takes the physician through a crafted tutorial on how to evoke a cure using the fundamental laws that he established.

The primary law of this modality is the "law of similars". This is based on the realization that the symptoms expressed by the patient are not the disease, but the positive reactions of the organism under stress in an attempt to regain physiological balance. The physician, in order to help the patient re-establish order, assists and strengthens these symptoms rather than suppresses or stifles them. The correct homeopathic remedy is selected based on its ability to produce those presenting symptoms in a healthy individual (accomplished through pain

---

[81] The Organon of the Art of Healing, 1810. Revised as 6 editions. The 6th edition was published well after his death in 1921. It contains 291 aphorisms. It is divided into a theoretical part and a section devoted to practice.

staking drug provings[82]). The ill patient will be extremely susceptible to that remedy, and his symptoms will be temporarily intensified in order to evoke a cure. Therefore, the same remedy that can produce those identical symptoms in the well individual, will heal the sick one.

What is Health according to homeopathy?

Health to a homeopath is harmony between all the different life processes of the body, a balance in the etheric body itself, the astral body and also between the two. The etheric and astral forces can, if they are unbalanced, create or restore an equilibrium by producing strong symptoms which quickly and efficiently remove any insult. A quick and high fever, for example, is a sign of a strong vital force. The object of giving a remedy that produces the same symptoms is to stimulate that vital force to initiate a curative response. This is in sharp contrast to allopathy, which views symptoms as the disease; consequently, symptoms are suppressed, and the vital force of the patient is compromised. Homeopathy does not prioritize disease as simply a result of pathogenic factors; nor does it view a cure as the simple removal of such factors.

The ultimate goal is more profound in nature. The inherit weaknesses of all living things, otherwise called susceptibility, must be sealed to insure a complete resolution of disease and optimal health. Brilliantly, Hahnemann artfully explained in the

---

[82] Proving: the term proving comes from the German word, Prüfung, which means to test. In homeopathy it is essential to test substances to find out which symptoms that substance is capable of producing, and thus curing. It is conducted on a group of volunteers who are in a good state of health, and who are not aware of the remedy that they are taking. The symptoms they experience are combined to create a total picture of the disease state the substance could be used for.

Organon what the physician was exactly trying to achieve; in other words, what constitutes health as stated in the following paragraph:

> *"In the healthy condition of man, the spiritual vital force, the dynamis that animates the material body (organism), rules with unbounded sway, and retains all the parts of the organism in admirable, harmonious, vital operation, as regards to both sensations and functions, so that one's in-dwelling, reason gifted mind can freely employ this living healthy instrument for the higher purpose of our existence"*

This paragraph is the first hint to the spiritual aspect of homeopathy and to the goal Hahnemann was trying to achieve. First, he actually refers to the vital force as a spiritual faculty bestowed upon life to animate the material world. Additionally, he refers to life as a gift from a higher force that also gave us free will (unbounded sway). And finally, the entire reason for the search for the holy grail of a cure; to fulfil our highest purpose. Not to simply procreate, breath, eat and survive, but to find our rightful spiritual essence as part of a larger cosmos.

If we compare our goal as a homeopath to the goal Dr. Thoresen sets out in this book, to achieve healing through the use of spiritual science, we discover that the goals are not only similar but complementary. As Hahnemann so clearly stated at the end of paragraph 9, the end goal is to facilitate freedom. For Dr Thoresen, as well as Rudolf Steiner, this freedom is achieved by the separation of the soul faculties of thinking, feeling and willing. George Vitoulkas, a widely renowned Greek homeopath paraphrased health as being a "freedom from pain in the physical body, from passion on the emotional level, having as a result a dynamic state of calm and serenity, and freedom from selfishness in the mental sphere, having as a result total unification with the truth". Therefore, health in homeopathy involves opening oneself up to the spiritual world with the end goal of being unified with the cosmic I representing all that exists.

In this regard, it is equally important that the homeopath immerses himself in the same idealism. Using his intellect to master his craft, but also maintain himself at the highest level of integrity, wisdom and love. As paragraph nine states, the physician wants to make people healthy so they can use their bodies for the higher purpose of their existence. It is my experience as a homeopath, that correct prescribing is a path to enable this goal, for both the homeopath administering the remedy and the patient receiving it.

What is the Similimum?

But the questions continue. Now that we understand our mission statement, how do we go about transforming the diseased so that they may fulfil such a purpose?

This can be found in Hahnemann's second law, which states that there is only one exact remedy at the time of administration that will evoke a curative response. This remedy is called the "similimum". At this point, Hahnemann focused on the individual. Every patient is treated as a unique being rather than a disease category. There is no remedy for diabetes, high blood pressure or a painful joint. We are not simply treating isolated symptoms. Instead we are looking at the stress strain model in its entirety. The way one organism reacts to a stressor will be completely different than another. In this way, we are evaluating the vital force of that unique being and it's concomitant susceptibility. This vital force is expressed through the symptoms that are not intended to be suppressed, but are used to drive healing. This expression is thus facilitated so that we are restored to permanent health, free to fulfil our higher purpose.

Hahnemann began exploring his theories by administering full strength extractions of various plants, animal and mineral substances to patients with acute diseases. He discovered that after an initial violent reaction, the diseased patient would recover fully. He later discovered that if he diluted the remedy in water and alcohol and succussed it (forcibly tapping the solution against a solid object), he actually excited the latent curative force of the substance and removed the physical toxicity. This process is known as potentization[83] and allowed the practitioner to reduce the initial aggravation and increase the effect on the patient's vital force.

Therefore, homeopathic treatment involves giving a patient with symptoms of illness extremely small doses of substances that produce the same symptoms in healthy people when given in larger doses. A homeopathic remedy is prepared by diluting the substance in a series of steps. Many homeopathic remedies are so highly diluted that no molecules of the original material substance are likely to remain.

The process of potentization developed into an organized nomenclature of specific strengths regarding remedy selection. It is almost as important to prescribe the level of potency administration as it is to select the similimum. If the potency is too low, the effect may be too weak to effect a change. However, if the potency is too strong, the patient's vital force may not be able to withstand the aggravation.

Hahnemann began with the weaker, X potencies or Decimal scale. The X signifies a dilution of 1:9, meaning that one part of the original remedy is added to 9 parts of alcohol and water. The resulting product is then successively succussed and diluted each time to create a potency. The X potencies are processed either 6

---

[83] Potentization: A much misunderstood fact about remedies is that they are diluted. Although the remedy is added to water, it is actually the process of potentization that creates the dynamic and altered effect of the remedy. This process is more like distillation where the aspects of the substance which remain are intensified by the process. Specifically, the material structure of the substances is diluted while its energetic aspect is magnified. In other words, potentized medicines are bridges between the physical and the spiritual.

or 12 times. The latter being the stronger remedy of the two. The label would then signify a 6x or a 12x potency. A stronger potency was then made by diluting one part to 99. This is called a C potency (C standing for centisimal). The most popular dilutions of the higher-powered C potencies are 30C which is diluted sequentially 1:99 for 30 times and 200C which is diluted 200 times. At the 200C level the remedy seems to take on exponentially more strength than the 30C, and therefore can create a more powerful reaction of the vital force. The next highest potency scale includes the M potencies. This is when the C potency has been diluted and succussed a 1000 times. It is signified by the label 1M. This is a very high potency. This remedy has also been diluted and succussed 10 and 50 more times to produce a 10M and 50M remedy.

Jeremy Scherer, a renowned Israeli homeopath, has a strong philosophy regarding potency prescription. He feels that the idea put forth by James Tyler Kent[84] that the higher the potency the more it affects the mental emotional plane is not totally accurate. We must view health as a highly dynamic level (unbounded sway). Therefore, a person in disease becomes more static. A dynamic patient needs a higher potency, therefore a scale from dynamic to static would be more accurate in order to determine potency. These dynamic qualities are found by looking at the modalities of a case (things that make the symptoms better or worse). Homeopaths often find that patients that are entering an incurable state have symptoms that can no longer be modulated, and therefore need smaller potencies. Other factors can include

---

[84] James Tyler Kent: a popular and famous American homeopath, who at the turn of the century advanced homeopathy into a highly influential philosophy formulated as a synthesis of mysticism and Christian religious ideology. Kent linked potentization to the ability to affect the spiritual world. He stated that all disease causes are invisible and nebulous, and all sickness originates from internal causes that are spiritual. As potentization and succession is a process that revives the material world, he. felt that the higher vibrational quality of higher potencies was a primary way to effect spiritual disease

the severity of the organic pathology, the poor lifestyle of the patient, the severity and number of mental disorders, and most importantly their sense of purpose and fulfilment. In the latter case, this would be a reason to give higher potencies as discussed by Kent.

How is the remedy Selected?

There are essential tools in the form of books, that are used by a homeopath for determining a remedy. The first book is a homeopathic '"Materia Medica"'. There are many of these books written by many authors, including both Hahnemann and Kent.

A "Materia Medica" is basically a record of the effects of active substances on healthy human beings. With the exception of Richard Pitcairn[85], a veterinarian from Oregon, and Dr. Milleman, a French veterinarian and homeopath, no thorough "Materia Medicas" have been written for animals. Homeopathic veterinarians extrapolate using the existing human "Materia Medicas" that have withstood the test of time.

Under each remedy a list of symptoms is categorized according to parts of the body effected (extremities, head, face, mental symptoms, etc.) and another category called Generalities. These are symptoms that effect the entire totality. I like to say they represent the "I" and not the "my", and because of this, develop a greater importance in determining the remedy. A generality may include phraseology such as "worse cold", "worse night", better with rest, etc.

Some "Materia Medicas" emphasize *key note* symptoms. These are symptoms that are strongly characteristic to that remedy. For

---

[85] New World Veterinary Repertory, Dr. Richard Pitcairn, Narayana pub, 2016. A prominent figure in veterinary classical homeopathy, began practicing homeopathy in 1986 and teaching this subject to veterinarians in 1992 in his hometown of Eugene, Oregon.

example, the remedy Phosphorus has the keynote symptom "fear of thunderstorms". Priority is given to both the generalities and the mental emotional state as both have a substantial effect on the entire being as expressed through the neuroendocrine axis. Hahnemann stated in the "Organon" that all disease begins with a sensation perceived first at the general and mental level. As one would guess, most "Materia Medicas" have been transcribed to computer software[86].

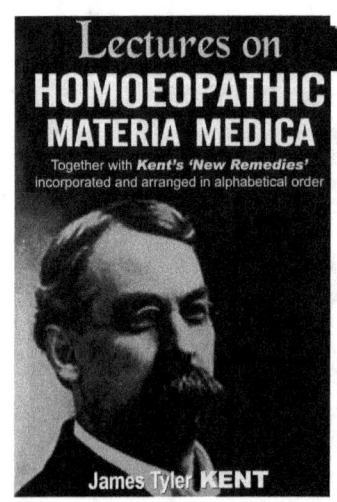

Detailed historical case taking is the cornerstone of successful prescribing. Most patients are afflicted with a complex layering of life long symptoms which reflect their reactions to a singular chronic disease pattern. The original weaknesses are meshed within complicated layers of morbid influences and suppressive allopathic medications which often forces the homeopath to prescribe first based on presenting symptoms. This aspect of case taking will become clearer as we discuss the concept of miasma in the next section.

---

[86] Homeopathic "Materia Medica"s on computer software: RadarOpus sold by Archibel and Macreperatory and Reference works sold by synergy homeopathic

Essentially, the homeopath records the pertinent symptoms and selects a remedy through the process called repertorization[87]. This will require the second major tool of the homeopath: a book called a repertory. This book catalogues all symptoms according to parts of the body. Each chapter covers an area of the patient; mind, extremities, bladder, chest, etc. Next to each symptom description, for example: mind, industrious, there will be a list of remedies that have that symptom as part of its makeup. These symptoms are discovered by medical provings and historical clinical observations.

Through a process of elimination, a selection of remedies arise that would elicit all the pertinent symptoms. As with the "Materia Medica", many repertories are also available and can be used as computer software. A list of relevant remedies are then compared and researched to determine which remedy represents the stress strain model of the patient. We will discuss how to analyse the list in the next section.

---

[87] Repertorization: The use of a lexicon of symptoms and their corresponding remedies to aid in the selection of an appropriate remedy based on detailed observations of the patients symptoms and medical history.

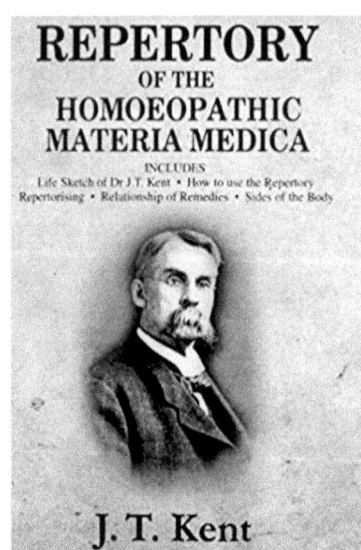

As long as the patient feels a global sense of improvement the remedy should never be repeated. The single most common error in prescribing is over medication. These remedies come in both pillules and liquid. The number of pillules in a single dose is less relevant than frequency of administration and, of course, potency.

Evaluation of a curative response: Hering's law of cure

In homeopathy, Hering's Law of Cure is widely recognized as Hahnemann's second law. Constance Hering was a medical physician and student of Hahnemann who, in 1845, published an essay called the *"Guide to the Progressive Development of Homeopathy"*. James Tyler Kent paraphrased this essay in his second lecture on homeopathic philosophy, where he stated that:

"A cure must proceed from center to circumference. From above downward, from within outwards, from more important to less important organs, from the head to the hands and the feet, and from recent symptoms to older ones"

Hering's Law of Cure is not theoretical. It is derived from repeated observations of homeopathic patients over many years. It has been verified time and again in clinical work through observations of patients as they move toward a cure.

Thus, in order to heal, one tends to undergo a definite and specific healing process, inner pathology needs to rise to the exterior before leaving the system entirely. Recent conditions must resolve before older more chronic conditions improve.

Healing can be uncomfortable at times, but understanding that the symptoms are following a reliable curative path can reassure the practitioner that the path is correct. In addition, knowing that suppressing symptoms, even for the short term, has a high probability of creating a deeper, more complicated problem in the long term. This can help to convince patients to make better choices regarding their health decisions.

Earlier in this text, Dr. Thoresen stated that Hering's law of cure does not represent the path of a cure. I would propose that actually it may not represent the *complete* path to a *final* cure, but rather the correct direction toward that cure. Thoresen was disturbed by the observation of the movement of the pathological entity from one part of the body to another, as if he was, through treatment, chasing an elusive parasite that is never truly annihilated (transformed). Although, I somewhat agree, I do not believe this is a random movement, but rather a movement toward exteriorization of serious illness to less essential areas. I would also propose that these symptoms may not be that of the original subversive force (i.e. demon) but the body's reaction to that subversive force. This would be similar to the measles pathogen (as would a demon) creating a vital force reaction of a rash just before the patient cures himself. Ultimately, Dr. Thoresen is correct if we consider the even higher definition of cure as a totality of cure of all living things. Therefore, ultimate cure should involve the "group" rather than the individual. In this context, Herings' laws do not extend beyond the exterior of that particular patient. As in measles, the patient is ultimately cured when the rash is exteriorized, but the contagion can still be passed to other members of the community. In this sense we are not truly curing the planet if we allow the subversive force to extend its illness to others.

Finally, as a homeopath, I believe there will always be subversive forces ready to invade a susceptible host, whether we call them viruses, bacteria or demons. For each demon exorcized by treating the middle, there will be others to enter the lines of a patient's susceptibility. I have already witnessed this repeatedly after group middle treatments performed by both Dr. Thoresen and myself. Despite the divine freeing of the patient from its demonic roommates, chronic disease seems, with time, to again rear its ugly head. The key still remains, in my humble opinion, to seal susceptibility. For this, we must understand more than possession. We must understand the origin of this susceptibility. Understanding Hahnemann's theory of chronic disease through the eyes of spiritual science may provide the answer.

Stress strain model and the vicious cycle of disease

A great illusion is the concept of a never-ending circle repeating itself. Never to allow growth to the future as a result of never looking back. A record stuck on the same groove, a dog chasing his tail until exhaustion, a hamster in a cage. We are stuck in a moment, devoid of choice and freedom. This represents the absence of the ultimate unbounded sway of health as stated by Hahnemann in paragraph 9 of the Organon.

We have already discussed the idea that symptoms are a strain to the stressors of life as a method to regain homeostasis. What if the stress strain model gets stuck? What if it becomes the only method to react to stress, only to be repeated in every circumstance that represents a threat? What if, in its reaction to the stress, the vital force overcompensates in its attempt to regain balance? And, finally, what if each time around the loop, the patient becomes less healthy and the cycle now becomes a downward spiral? This is the description of chronic disease. The ultimate Groundhog Day.

Each patient has his own cycle of pathology represented by his own individual reaction to stress. To create a cycle, it has to begin somewhere. We could, for example, use the chief complaint. We could put it into the language of a simple phrase such as weakness. Under that category we could place exhaustion, weakness in the knees, blurry vision and so on. The next step is to understand what makes this weakness. This leads one to the modalities of aggravation. Perhaps discharges such as diarrhoea, menses or even yelling. On the flip side of the chief complaint would be the modalities that make it better (in homeopathic terminology, amelioration). Perhaps the patient improves with resting, applying warmth, meditating, or eating. Eventually this will lead the patient to the opposite side of the cycle of weakness; perhaps a sense of fullness, or a sense of having too much. This will then lead to other ameliorating modalities such as a desire to move, in other words, to discharge. This then brings us back to the beginning of the cycle, which is weakness. With this model, we can then select and categorize each symptom that is relative to the thread of the case. With this tool, we can readily see the emergence of two polar opposites with a set of modalities setting these opposites apart as the pendulum swings from one side to the other. This model allows us to look at the big picture, in other words, the entire story of the person. Like all good stories, we can remember it and access it easily to find the appropriate remedy that matches that cycle of pathology.

A good example of this process would be to understand the state that a person is in when they need the remedy "carcinosum", a remedy derived from breast cancer cells. The reader should be advised, that homeopathy is not isopathy. The remedy is never used as an exact product of the disease to be annihilated. This goes against the homeopathic principle of treating the totality

Interestingly, most carcinosum patients do not present with cancer, but it is often found in their relatives. In essence, patients needing carcinosum often present with fear and anxiety that creates a need to be taken care of by others (segment of fear). Because they have submitted their will (being taken care of) they lose their sense of self and go inward. As they are being cared for, they feel the walls close in on them and they begin to submissively resent the control over their life. Now we see the opposite happen, the over attention aggravates. Finally, they break out. This breaking out can appear as a twitch, or they develop other various discharges, and they can even become a bit self-destructive. Now, this frenzied activity leads to a breakdown such as ulcers, osteoporosis, and other forms of weakness. Finally, they are weakened, become fearful and as a result they look to be taken care of again.

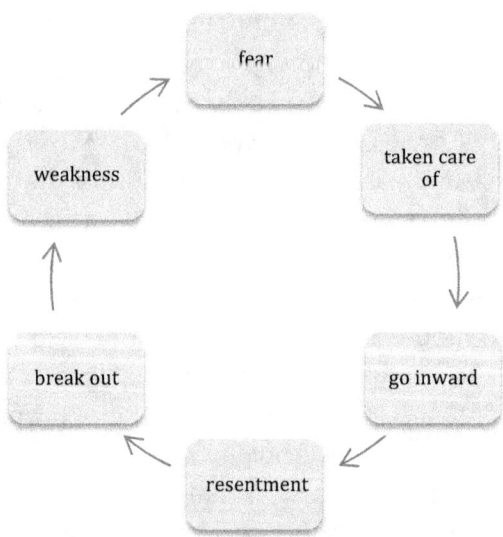

Cycle of Carcinosum

If one thinks about cancer, it is essentially a giving up of an organ function to become the invading organ. Ultimately this kind of loss of identity leads to self-destruction. The self-destruction leads to hospice and being taken care of and losing one's "self". It has been found that many children of cancer parents or grandparents will need this remedy at some point in their life.

As Dr. Thoresen described earlier, when he discussed the attributes of Ahriman and Lucifer, he compared them as yin and yang opposites. He described Ahriman as the fundamental pathological substance of yin while the Luciferic qualities are that of yang. He also noted that if the distance between the two demons is far apart within the midsection of the patient, the host is healthier. As the demons join together, chronic disease moves toward incurability as seen with terminal cancer. Using the perspective of a homeopath, this merging is characterized by a lack of modalities. If one analyses the cycle in cycles and segments, he will find that the modalities represent the segments that keep the two demons separated. Thus, cancer thrives when modalities no longer exist. This is a known observation among homeopaths as a marker of incurability.

This is exactly what cancer is; the loss of individuality. The giving up of the female and male individuality to become amorphous. Similar to the appearance of the internal organs of advanced cancer patients, as each individual cell is no longer recognizable. This exemplifies the causative factor of cancer (as explained earlier by Dr Thoresen) as a misunderstanding between man (yang) and woman (yin). This remedy cycle represents, at a demonic level, what is happening in the patient.

Demonology as a causative factor in homeopathy

However, the homeopathic doctrine cannot be fully understood as long as there is not a clear understanding of the operation of the vital force of the patient in regard to spirituality. This was discussed in Hahnemann's book, "The Theory of Chronic

Disease".[88] The tenants of classical homeopathy state that there are two types of creative forces, harmonic and subversive. The former is vital for the normal functions and development of the body while the latter produces those substances in nature that are adapted to the organism in disturbance. Both forces, by their action upon matter, embody themselves in visible forms. The results which these forces create by their action upon matter are united to those forces by that same indivisible bond which unites effect to cause.

The answer seemed simple. One must introduce the natural form of existence of that variety of subversive force which has invaded the organism. These types being united to the forces by that indivisible bond shown to exist between effect and cause, the disease will of its own accord leave the organism which is not its natural product or type and embody itself in its natural type which is the medicinal substance. This is the same way a ray of sun converges in the focus of a burning glass.

Hahnemann had more questions. By what process, and in what manner does the invasion of the organism by the subversive forces take place and disease constituted. He stated that any answer to that was speculative reasoning. However, if one was to read these statements regarding subversive forces they could easily come to the conclusion that these are the demons mentioned throughout this book.

---

[88] The Theory of Chronic disease: written in 1828 by Samuel Hahneman at the age of 73. This book was his redemption for failing to cure patients with his previous methods. He writes about the miasms as unknown exterior agents that were causing an obstacle to cure. These dynamic conceptions were quite different and more complex than the material pathogens of conventional medicine. There remained hidden diseases not visible and not treatable by his prior homeopathic system of treatment.

The Theory of Chronic Disease and the concept of "Miasm".

Although Hahnemann enjoyed great success in the treatment of acute diseases, by 1816, he started to doubt his modality. He was discovering that despite his best efforts, the health of his patients seemed to be slowly declining. As he agonized over this deterioration in his patients, he began fervently searching for a deeper understanding of the processes that lie behind chronic disease. He wrote the following, regarding his chronically diseased patients, "*their beginning was promising, the continuation less favourable, the outcome hopeless.*" As he continued to administer his remedies he noticed that certain chronic patients, who responded well at first, either relapsed or slowly became more ill. Of this experience, he said:

> "*The remedy which was serviceable the first time would prove less useful, and when repeated again it would help still less*".

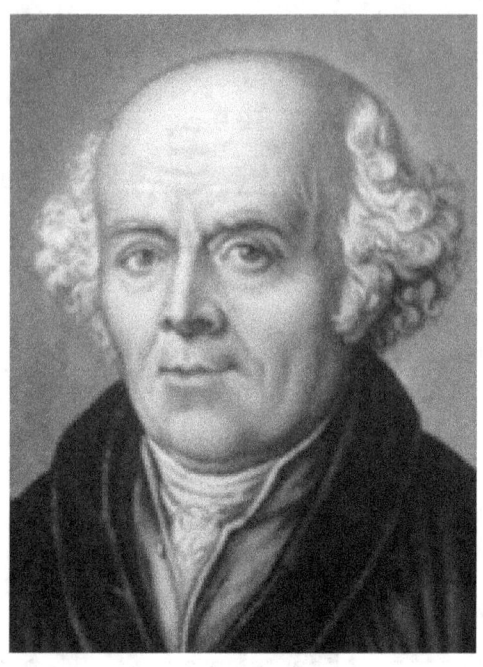

Samuel Hahnemann   April 10, 1755 – July 2, 1843

As Hahnemann watched these patients closely, he noticed that new symptoms would be added to the old ones that could be removed only "inadequately and imperfectly". Again, despite prescribing an appropriate remedy, each dose became less effective and in the end, they worked "no better than weak palliatives". This left him more determined to find the cause of this resistance.

For over a decade Hahnemann secretly searched for the reason for his failures. Finally, in 1828 he presented his findings in the first edition of his great work, *The Chronic Diseases*. Over the next 11 years he produced 4 more editions of this work that were published in 1830, 1835, 1837 and 1839. This work was followed in 1839 by the 4th edition of the *Organon*. In these works, Hahnemann made public for the first time his theory of the chronic *miasms*. This marks the first major divide since the conception of homeopathy. With the introduction of the theory of Psora and the chronic miasms, many of his followers believed that he had gone too far. They felt more comfortable with what Hahnemann had practiced in his earlier years. He was well aware that his new ideas were controversial, and shortly before the publication of his findings, he wrote to a colleague the following:

> *"They will require more than six months before they recover from the fright and astonishment of this enormous, preposterous affair and will perhaps need another six months before they will believe in it. Therefore, it will probably be three years before they can make any sensible use of it".*

For me, the most fascinating aspect of Hahnemann's journey is the way it parallels the author's path toward writing this book. Having the honour of being his student for 30 years I have witnessed Thoresen's almost identical suffering. The rewriting of books, the eventual demise of his cancer treatment, and finally the discovery of a deeper and more profound understanding. And with this better way, has come controversy. It is as if his "demon theory" has mirrored Hahnemann's "miasmatic theory".

The simple fact is that Hahnemann, as all physicians, wanted to understand what caused chronic disease. Hippocrates taught that all diseases were caused by the predisposition inherent in the innate constitution. In the *Organon of Medicine,* in Aphorism 5, Hahnemann divided the origin of disease into two categories, the exciting and fundamental causes, and related them very closely, as did Hippocrates, to the susceptibility of the physical constitution. Here is where we first hear of the idea of a miasm:

> *"Useful to the physician in assisting him to cure are the particulars of the most probable exciting cause of the acute disease as well as the most significant points in*

> the complete history of the chronic disease, to enable him to discover its fundamental cause, which is generally due to a chronic miasm. In these investigations, the ascertainable physical constitution of the patient (especially when the disease is chronic), his moral and intellectual character, his occupation, mode of living and habits, his social and domestic relations, his age, sexual function, etc., are to be taken into consideration".

This is where Hahnemann also makes a distinction between an acute self-limiting condition created by an epidemiological and overwhelming pathogen (Luciferic entity) and a deep-seated chronic disease (Ahrimanic entity). Acute diseases are illnesses, which have quick onsets, rapid progressions, and an ultimate resolution to death or cure. In this transient state the constitutional condition is temporarily suppressed and the overall picture is changed. However, many of these acute diseases are actually acute exacerbations of the chronic states latent within the constitution that have been brought forth by exciting factors (Ahriman inviting Lucifer in). Here, the patients overall general constitutional state still remains unchanged. The nature of this chronic miasmic disease is slow and insidious in its onset and gradual in its progression. These negative transformations gradually increase until they bring on complex pathologies that eventually are the cause of premature old age and death. These chronic miasms are the effects of subversive forces that are not self-limiting, and cause considerable damage to the immune system, the vital force, and the constitution.

What is a Miasm?

Depiction of a Miasm by Robert Seymour

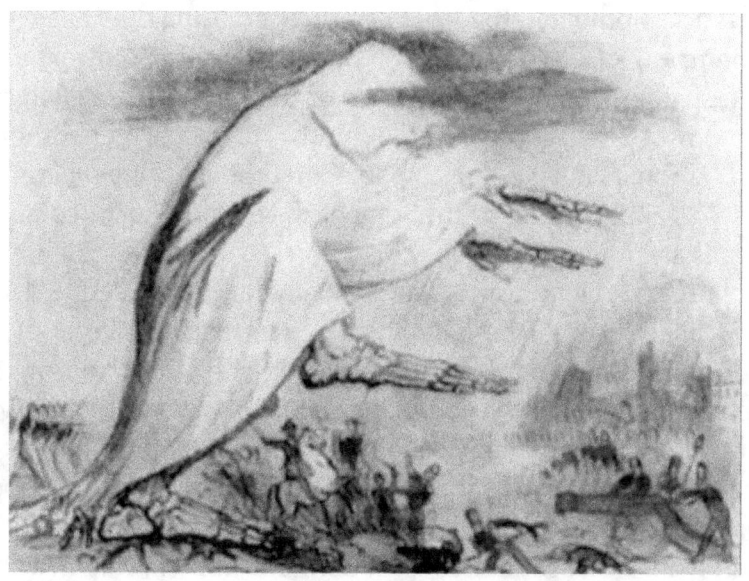

The word Miasm originates in Greek mythology. It represents a contagious power that has an independent life force of its own, and, until purged, society would be chronically infected by catastrophe as a result of its influence. For most physicians, it has come to represent the germ theory. As such, the word pollutant or contagion became equal to infectious disease. However, Hahnemann had a special and deeper understanding of the word miasm. For him, it is understood to be a derangement of the vital force that predates and is more fundamental than the current illness the patient suffers from. In addition, this dynamic malady inflicts itself upon large groups of humanity and remains from generation to generation creating common and unchanging characteristics that remain impregnated in those afflicted. Therefore, according to Hahnemann, it is the job of the physician to try to understand the whole of the true disease inside the patient, not just what is currently perceived. To do so, he must find out as far as possible, the whole extent of all the accidents and symptoms belonging to this unknown "primitive malady."

In Classical Homoeopathy (that as practiced using the tenants of Hahnemann), the word "miasm" means the effects of external subversive forces on the vital force of the patient, including the symptoms that are transmitted to the following generations. These chronic miasms are capable of producing degenerative illnesses, and can lead the organism toward such complex diseases as immuno-deficiency disorders.

The three chronic miasms that Hahnemann introduced in 1828 were called Psora (the itch miasm, Ahrimanic), Sycosis (the gonorrhoeal miasm, Luciferic) and Syphilis (the cancer miasm, the cooperation between Ahriman and Lucifer). A fourth miasm was later added by Hahnemann called "The tubercular miasm".

According to the founders of Homeopathy, to overlook Hahnemann's doctrine of chronic disease is to miss the importance of causation, constitution, and the chronic miasms. This trinity forms the foundation of the concept of the totality of the signs and symptoms. Hahnemann classified some remedies into anti-miasmic categories because he discovered that certain deep acting medicines have a similar nature to the syndromes produced by the miasms. James Tyler Kent stated in his treatise on observing the patient:

> "A great deal depends upon a physician's ability to perceive what constitutes the miasm. If he is dull of perception, he will intermingle symptoms that do not belong together, Hahnemann seems to have had the most wonderful perception, he seemed to see at a glance."

What Kent discovered, simply stated, is that complex disease is often made up of many interdependent components rather than one constitutional factor. It takes a series of related remedies to remove the miasmatic layers as the patient moves toward health. It is important to then know in what order the layers of the case have formed along the timeline so that they may be unraveled in the reverse order by which they developed.

What do these miasms look like?

Each chronic miasm has its own characteristic signs that are a part of the totality or the cycle we discussed above. For example, Psora has the main feature of weakness and hypo function. Often the skin will play a strong role in pathogenesis along with problems in digestion and the eliminative organs. It is theorized that psora is actually the original sin representing the weakness of man's free will analogized by the Bible's Garden of Eden. In acupuncture, this would represent the symptoms of a Qi deficiency. In the anthroposophical world, it manifests in the soul faculty of will and at the level of the I consciousness. In actuality, this miasm represents the original constitution of the patient rather than the effect of a subversive force.

The sycotic miasm tends to exhibit symptoms of excess and overgrowth. In acupuncture, the description would be analogous to diseases of a yang nature. In anthroposophy, it reflects the soul faculty of feeling and acts at the level of the astral body.

Syphilitic miasms are degenerative, going toward an internalized self-destruction of the patient. In acupuncture, these diseases would be under the category of yin, representing the soul faculty of thinking and effecting the etheric.

The reader should be asking why these miasms are named after major disease categories. If one looks at pathogens from the view point of a homeopath, he must approach this question with the concept that pathogens are the opportunists of a poorly developed soil. The miasm represents the susceptibility of the subversive force, and that susceptibility allows the overgrowth of pathogens that have an affinity for the descriptions written above. Gonorrhoea, a sycotic disease is represented by the development of fig warts as overgrowths from attracting these types of venereal contagions. These yang types tend to find themselves traveling the seven seas only to return home with a host of invasive pathogens to spread to the next sycotic individual. The susceptibility occurs before the pathogenic factors invade.

Syphilis is a much more serious and fatal venereal disease. Its affinity is toward ulceration and decay and attacks the bone, nervous system and teeth. These patients tend toward a singular lifestyle, with melancholy and possible suicide.

Hahnemann's newer Tubercular miasm, concomitant with the appearance of Tuberculosis (as its name implies) tends to target the chest, particularly the lung. The temperament tends toward romantic longing with an optimistic yet dissatisfied state that lends itself to constant change.

Using this information, it is important for the homeopath to determine which miasm is predominating at the moment of treatment. Most often these miasms are representative of an obstacle to true cure. The ultimate goal is to clear the path for the use of an antipsoric. The homeopath is now able to ultimately cure the original sin that started with the weakness of will. There are a host of remedies that predominate in each category. They are found in the reparatory under the headings of their names in the category titled *generalities*.

To add a final category, it has been surmised by some that cancer is now a newer miasm that is actually a combination of the other miasms. It is interesting to note that Thoresen has already mentioned that cancer occurs when Ahriman and Lucifer join together. This is a hint to the next theory that we shall discuss.

The idea that these miasms are representative of the demons of anthroposophic medicine.

Are miasms demons?

In order to begin this discussion, we have to come to the conclusion that within the spiritual world there are both good and evil forces. These evil forces or demons are prolific, to the point that it appears that all of mankind is infected. With this understanding, we as healers must take seriously the arduous task of not only understanding the purpose of these beings in relationship to mankind, but our purpose in creating a global cure through their transformation.

We should start with the actual definition of a demon as it relates to healing. As mentioned in earlier chapters, Demons are those entities of the spirit world that exist in the material world as pathological structures with their own life force. In other words, they have a sinister effect upon humans by feeding off the negative emotions and thoughts of their host. In fact they cannot thrive without this source of energy. Another source of energy is the Karmic web called by many the geopathic influence[89].

In anthroposophy, the two sides of man are viewed as being a balance or fight between Luciferic and Ahrimanic powers, where Lucifer is the masculine and Ahriman the feminine power. Lucifer represents the left side and Ahriman the right. But even though they are seen as evil powers, they are necessary factors in our development, as we not only need the feminine and masculine influence, we need to find the balance between them.

---

[89] More about this subject in part two of this trilogy

Demons as Miasms

As mentioned earlier, Demons originally were of a good nature, as a creation of the actions of other higher beings. However, at some point, they did not continue to participate in the cosmic evolution. The Luciferic demon remained behind and incarnated into the human body in the third millennium before Christ. The Ahrimanic force descended to the depths of the earth's core and reincarnated after Christ. At this point Ahriman, also known as Satan, became much more sinister. In this way they developed their synonyms, Lucifer being the light spirit while Ahriman became that of the dark. Both bring their delusions with them as they enter mankind. Lucifer, as the light bearer, brings delusions of divinity, creativity, and spirituality that are at a heightened state of development, but accompanied by a complete denial of the material world. In contrast, Ahriman's delusion is denial of the spiritual world, accompanied by a high level of intellectual prowess, a strong avarice, and a love of technology and money.

As man became disconnected from the spirit world, lured by the desires and cravings of the material, a sort of susceptibility or weakness was created. This susceptibility allowed entry for these subversive forces to thrive. Their desire is to dominate and entangle the soul faculties of man to serve their own unique purposes. A spiritual battle is being fought at this current time with Ahriman in the forefront.

One might conclude that the attributes of both forces, at a certain level, are helpful for the continued evolution of mankind, but the demonic part of these forces, created or let in by the amoral actions of man, is to be considered evil. Therefore, demons should not be regarded as either pure evil or pure goodness. It is therefore not the job of the healer to annihilate them, but as both Steiner and Thoresen state, redirect them toward a balance between both attributes so as to serve their higher purpose in helping us rather than creating harm. The same goal stated in paragraph 9, that of freeing ourselves so that we can follow our higher purpose, is not just for us but the demons that serve as our obstacles to cure. Of course, this is accomplished through Christ's love as exemplified by treating the middle, or as I hope to prove, the correct homeopathic remedy prescription.

The Attributes of Ahriman and Lucifer.

In Traditional Chinese Medicine, the world is divided into two polarities. Yin is representative of the female energy. It is dark and cool like a winter's night. Its energy is subdued and its disease state tends toward deficiency. It's polar opposite, yang, represents male energy; hot and bright, and full of activity. As such, it's disease state leans toward excess. With this in mind, we can easily categorize Lucifer as representing the yang excess state and Ahriman representing that of yin deficiency.

Lucifer manifests with hyperactivity. The energy is frenzied often bordering on a mania. It tends to create a fantasy world, filled with many illusions and creating a world of phobias. The sympathetic nervous system qualities of flight or fight are exaggerated, and as such, solace is found in the safety of the tribe as unification becomes an adaptation to such a state. Although highly flexible, it can lack rigidity and substance creating a sense of being outside of the body. Without a clear recognition of earthly matters, it sees eating and drinking as a necessity, often forgotten. The spirit world is its only desire, and as such, it delves so much in such matters that it develops a false illusion that it is of great divinity. Often the singular belief in Christ consciousness is lost as the scattered energy of this force is spread among too many false belief systems.

Ahriman on the other hand, is reflective of the yin. Unlike the hyperactive exuberance of Lucifer, this force is subdued, bordering on tedium. It favors organization and structure over impulsivity. So much so, that rigidity replaces flexibility. The ultimate sceptic, Ahriman, denies the existence of anything that cannot be proven or measured. This force goes so far in this realm that it actually has a tendency to worship the quantitative aspects of materialism. Greed and avarice dominate. These material possessions are obtained by the current dedication to technology. This dogmatic and intellectual type craves the cold deductive logic that is the necessity of creating such inventions. In its desire to accrue material possessions, this type will store things beyond what is necessary with an underlying anxiety regarding poverty. This rigid stance can appear in the physical form as rigidity of the joints as well as the brain. Science becomes his God. Even if he takes up religion it is performed in such a ritualistic and intellectual fashion that the words are taken too literally.

The Cycles of Lucifer and Ahriman

Lucifer
1. sensitive, clairvoyant, sees beyond the material world, connects with all
2. feels overwhelmed, too many sensations too many feelings .. too full
3. discharge ... frenzied activity
4. spends energy which scatters him, loses sense of self, stops eating, leaves body
5. intense fear and phobias
6. suppresses and hardens which leads to a need to express
7. seeks company for reassurance, needs to unify

Summary of the Luciferic cycle: Sensitive to the environment and to the feelings and sounds of the spirit world...makes him overwhelmed with the sensations...makes activity frenzied .... creates a big discharge, disintegrates, and loses sense of his body...this makes him fearful and panicky which makes him seek company. However, the company makes him over sensitive to the feelings of those he seeks.

Ahriman
1. Rigid and inflexible
2. Sensitive to disorder
3. Desires clear boundaries and definitions
4. Needs material
5. Fear of loss, poverty
6. Isolates and hides

Summary of the Ahrimanic cycle: rigidity leads to an intolerance for disorder. This then leads for a strong desire for laws and concrete material things which leads to a fear of losing those things. This makes him hide and isolate from others, even to the point of hurting others in order to maintain his rigid life style.

With the clearly emerging totality of sycosis (Lucifer) and syphilis (Ahriman) as presented as repeating cycles, the task now is to find which remedies in the "Materia Medica" can be adapted to the healing of the 4-fold view of man as seen in Anthroposophy.

The reader should keep in mind that the transformation of Lucifer and Ahriman does not result in the ultimate cure but rather a removal of a strong insurmountable obstacle to cure. Dr. Thoresen has discovered, through the use of an acupuncture needle to treat the middle, that he can remove these demons from the patient. More importantly, he has discovered the true power in adding group therapy that leads the individual to the unity of mankind, which is in essence the ultimate goal of our existence. It is in this way that the demons are not only removed, but transformed into beneficial entities

For those not versed in the use of acupuncture and even more important, not developed in their spiritual senses, Homeopathy may provide an alternative method in removing such obstacles. In classical homeopathy, medorrhinum represents the main remedy that exemplifies sycosis, while syphilinum was the original remedy mentioned for the syphilitic state. Listed below are the cycles for these two remedies:

Medorrhinum(sycotic miasm) The equivalence to Lucifer

1. excessive desire to connect with others
2. discharge (frenzied activity)
3. burned out and debilitated
4. Scattered and spaced out, lives outside the body
5. Fear of outside influences coming in, fear of internal impulses
6. Try to suppress themselves by hardening
7. This hardening builds and traps energy inside that needs to be expressed to others as desires

When comparing this cycle to the one of Lucifer, there is a strikingly similar pattern of pathology.

Syphilinum (syphilitic miasm) the equivalence to Ahriman

1. Fear that they will be killed or robbed, world is hostile
2. to limit the threat, they control themselves and their world
3. develop compulsive and complex ritualistic behaviours for safety to prevent bad things from happening
4. Feel antisocial and separate which keeps the person alone

5. feel like they are going crazy because of their compulsions
6. they then try to break through and connect but this leads to 1.

As with Ahriman, there is a strong desire to create order and boundaries in order to protect themselves and the material possessions that they so strongly desire. As mentioned above, historically, these two remedies, Medorrhinum for Sycosis, and Syphilinum for Syphilis, have been the representative for these two major miasms. However, if one looks at the "Materia Medica" chapter entitled generalities, Sycosis and Generalities, syphilis there are many remedies that fall under each category.

If we take into consideration the concepts of the 4 levels of the human organism, however, we may realize that a true cure might only be achieved by working at the very deepest layer of the human existence, at what is called the I or ego level. This reflects the deepest level of the law of cure, the level that goes beyond Kent's concept of emphasizing mentals and generalities. These concepts can be only understood by exploring the tenants of anthroposophic medicine.

Classical Homeopathy vs Anthroposophic Medicine

Steiner's major tool in his search for medical approaches to human suffering was centered around his unique ability to perceive the spiritual world. Using the basic concepts of Goethe,[90] which he

---

[90] **Johann Wolfgang von Goethe** (August 28, 1749 – March22, 1832) was a German writer and statesman. His works included prose, dramas; memoirs; treatises on botany, anatomy, and colour; and four novels. In addition, numerous literary and scientific fragments, more than 10,000 letters, and nearly

edited in his early years, and the use of anthroposophic meditation, he described the dynamics of the living material world as the result of three interacting systems of life forces. Besides the material body, this would include the etheric body which controls the material bodies formative forces, the astral body which controls the experience of life as inner emotions, and finally, the concept of ego (the I) and self-consciousness (a process unique to man).

3,000 drawings by him exist. A literary celebrity by the age of 25, Goethe was ennobled by the Duke of Saxe-Weimar, Carl August in 1782 after taking up residence there in November 1775 following the success of his first novel, *The Sorrows of Young Werther*. His first major scientific work, the *Metamorphosis of Plants*, was published after he returned from a 1788 tour of Italy. In 1791, he was made managing director of the theatre at Weimar, and in 1794 he began a friendship with the dramatist, historian, and philosopher Friedrich Schiller, whose plays he premiered until Schiller's death in 1805. During this period, Goethe published his second novel, *Wilhelm Meister's Apprenticeship*, the verse epic *Hermann and Dorothea*, and, in 1808, the first part of his most celebrated drama, *Faust*.

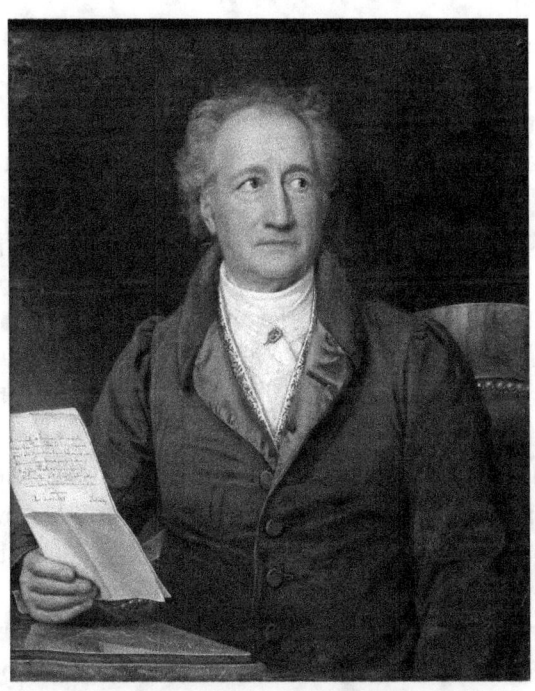

Johann Wolfgang von Goethe

Therefore, according to Steiner, health must be seen and understood from the aspect of these spiritual levels encasing the physical. In disease, these levels will be out of balance and therefore the therapist must find the substance that can restore health among all four levels. Constitutionally speaking, this ultimately refers to prioritizing the "I" or ego level, which, I feel, represents the original Psora. Psora, in this context, represents the free will of man to make decisions regarding good and evil. Anthroposophy states that these decisions include not just the individual but entire civilizations and are carried through the generations as "Karma". This Karma is equivalent to the weakness in all of mankind that allowed the susceptibility to original disease. This is in stark contrast to classical homeopathy, which focuses more on the vital force, which is observed only in the physical-etheric-astral relationship.

Secondly, Steiner continued to divide living organisms into three physiological processes that, at a spiritual level, maintain the soul faculties of thinking, feeling, and willing. He named these processes the poles. The first center is the cephalic pole controlling the brain, nervous system and skeleton. This pole harmonizes the soul faculty of thinking. The second center is dubbed the metabolic pole. This is the most active pole and includes circulation, blood, muscles and all physical activity. These processes allow correct functioning of the will. Finally, the third center is called the rhythmic pole which controls the organs of homeostasis such as the lungs, heart, kidney, pancreas and endocrine organs, thus providing the physiological basis of feeling. These three systems are the basis for Steiner's classification of illness. Inflammatory conditions, for example are caused by over activity of the metabolic pole. It is interesting to note that the redness of the metabolic pole is contrasted against the pale cold whiteness of the cephalic pole. He saw balance in the treatment of opposite poles. He also employed the idea of the "signature" in deciding appropriate remedies[91]. The whiteness of the cephalic pole resembles calcium, chalk and limestone while the redness of the metabolic pole points to iron, rust, and sulphur. In addition, if the cephalic pole represents the brain and nervous system, a homeopath might see the reasoning of employing such neurotrophic agents as the phosphates, natrums, and mercury. If one also includes the bone involvement with this pole, other remedies would include the allium family such as calcarea flourica, calcarea phosphorica, and the silicates. Steiner's heavy reliance on signatures in nature explains his use of different compounds which overlaps the concepts of constitutions in classical

---

[91]https://www.komplettapotek.no/kampanje/13733/weleda?gclid=Cj0KCQjwn ubLBRC_ARIsAASsNNm_X-Lopez5CHi-UkglB8jaWjTUkO2PPe2SRDMFZUO0qAk4_E0xvmMaAtROEALw_wcB

homeopathy. A perfect example is his discussion on the remedy Silicea. Silicea can be found in the detail of mollusc shells and as such Steiner surmised that Silicea types can have lovely features with delicate hair and skin. If one looks at the delicate branching growths that occur when silicate crystals are formed, ananthroposophist postulates that this observation might be representative of the delicacy and fineness of the Silica drug picture. Hahnemann, however, played down or dismissed the importance of the doctrine of signatures as a method for finding remedies and preferred the scientific principles and accuracy of his detailed provings. For Steiner, his doctrine was more subtle and complex than literal interpretations suggest and as such, required more depth of contemplation of a plant, drug, or body-part in order to penetrate its full metaphysical significance.

It appears that hindsight demonstrates a large chiasma between classical homeopathy and anthroposophic medicine in both approach and philosophy. In fact, the only resemblance to homeopathy in AM is the idea of dilution. Hahnemann's provings often revealed the doctrine of signatures in his provings, but it certainly was not the basis for finding the similimum. Pulsatilla, for example, is also called the yellow flower and provings have shown that the discharges of a pulsatilla illness are yellow in nature. Steiner had no "Materia Medicas of anthroposophic medicine, and he could not make sense of the homeopathic classical "Materia Medicas" of the day. He saw every symptom in every remedy. He quotes, "*The scrutiny of homeopathic medicine does not always furnish satisfactory results. Homeopathy attempts to handle the human being as a whole as it forms a comprehensive picture of all the symptoms and attempts to build a bridge to therapy. But in despair I find the remedies enumerated one after another and recommended for an entire legion of illnesses, everything beneficial for so much.*" His frustration is a common theme in homeopathy when one does not understand the true meaning of the concept of totality. This crucial point that eluded him has been only recently explained coherently by the concept of segments and cycles as explained above.

The other difference between homeopathy and the remedies of anthroposophy is that the latter are prepared in complex ways and are often combined with many substances. They are directed at the disturbance of the organ poles and the spiritual level of the disease, rather than the totality of the patient's stress-strain model. Their names reveal what organs their treatments target. Hepatodoron, Cardiodoran and Digestodoron are examples of such combinations and sold by a singular company by the name of Weleda. Anthroposophists claim to see every illness from its individual manifestation, yet justify such wide ranging basic remedies when disorders are considered to be the result of a combined destiny and the nature of modern age and civilization. These disorders then affect many people similarly and as such, medicines are often used for typical classifications of disease. This is in sharp contrast to classical homeopathy that never labels disease as a thing to be treated but rather the reaction of the individual's vital force as a stress-strain model.

There are, however, fundamental similarities that allows one to bridge and even merge their apparently disparate remedy selections. First, both modalities seek to look at the patient in terms of the totality. For homeopathy, it is to take every symptom pertinent to the stress strain model of the patient and use it to find a remedy that would elicit this stress strain model in a healthy being. For anthroposophy, the totality would include all 4 levels of mankind, meaning the physical, etheric, astral and I. In both modalities, mankind has developed several obstacles to cure that have invaded the human organism as a kind of subversive force. For homeopathy, these are the miasms of syphilis, sycosis, and cancer. For Anthroposophic Medicine, these are the symptoms of Ahriman, Lucifer, and Azuras. For Homeopathy, these miasms represent an assault on large groups of people and are passed on from generation to generation, and for Anthroposophic medicine, the diseases arise from the understanding of man's karmic destiny that is equally global in its scope, working at a level beyond the astral level of homeopathic remedies. This is the "I" level.

The marriage of homeopathy and anthroposophy.

To summarize the discussion above, one must appreciate the importance of Anthroposophic Medicine in the treatment of patients using the middle point and group therapy. The middle point is a way of activating the highest level of healing at the "I" or ego level. The straight uprightness reflected in the supreme health of man represents an uncompromising ability to stay centred in all three dimensions. This would apply to the activation of an energetic core middle. Anthroposophic literature implies that at a metaphysical level, this centre reflects a thin membrane along the length of the sternum, skull and abdomen that, in pathology, is weakened. This weakness prevents uprightness and also allows for the merging of Luciferic with Ahrimanic forces. This weakened "I" is another way of saying a weakened will. In homeopathy, this is referred to as the weakened state of Psora.

Therefore, we can assume that, in order to combine homeopathy with anthroposophic medicine, we must overlap those anthroposophic remedies that treat the "I" with the antipsoric remedies of classical homeopathy. This allows treatment at all levels of existence, both spiritually and materially and both individually as well as globally.

It is important to also understand the importance of first removing the fundamental obstacles to cure found in the presence of the subversive forces that have parasitized mankind since the beginning of time. In Anthroposophic Medicine they are seen as demonic evil entities that keep man in the delusion of illness. In Classical homeopathy, they are called miasms and have been termed according to the symptoms they portray which underscores the greater scope of pathologies than for which they are named. For Dr Thoresen, the removal of these subversive forces lies in strengthening the middle in order to "disarm them".

In homeopathy, the obstacles are removed by the use of miasmatic remedies. Once the pathogenic factors have been removed, a curative reaction can be then be achieved by the use of the remedies that will be explained in the next section.

The antipsorics of classical homeopathy

As was discussed earlier, Psora represents the "original disease". This is man's original fall from grace resulting in the fear and shame that created the material world with the idea of a body that can experience a sensation[92]. Correcting the Karma of suffering might be achieved in homeopathy by the ultimate use of the antipsoric remedies listed by Hahnemann.

The Psoric state can be summarized in a single word "weakness". In anthroposophical terms, this would be those states representing a weakness of the soul faculty of willing. In homeopathy, there is a constellation of symptoms that would imply such a weakness which can also be mirrored at a kind of deficiency state in the mental, emotional and physical levels.

---

[92] 3:1 Now the serpent was more subtle than any beast of the field which Jehovah God had made. And he said unto the woman, Yea, hath God said, Ye shall not eat of any tree of the garden? 3:2 And the woman said unto the serpent, Of the fruit of the trees of the garden we may eat: 3:3 but of the fruit of the tree which is in the midst of the garden, God hath said, Ye shall not eat of it, neither shall ye touch it, lest ye die. 3:4 And the serpent said unto the woman, Ye shall not surely die: 3:5 for God doth know that in the day ye eat thereof, then your eyes shall be opened, and ye shall be as God, knowing good and evil. 3:6 And when the woman saw that the tree was good for food, and that it was a delight to the eyes, and that the tree was to be desired to make one wise, she took of the fruit thereof, and did eat; and she gave also unto her husband with her, and he did eat. 3:7 And the eyes of them both were opened, and they knew that they were naked;

Symptoms of psora at a mental and emotional level often manifests as anxiety, particularly regarding anticipation, worry over health, and a fear of being alone. Such worry can eventually lead to exhaustion. Physically, psora manifests as a tendency toward skin disorders with itching, nutritional problems such as malabsorption, and numerous functional disturbances. The patient tends to be worse during the day and better resting.

To understand the general cycle of psora, we can look at its nosode, psorinum.

Psorinum Cycle:

1. Emptiness and sense of loss (weakness)
2. Creates anxiety
3. Creates a strong desire for things and people
4. Acquires so much they erupt
5. Then develops a disgust and aversion for the things they have
6. Gets rid of all their stuff...skin eruptions, job, divorce

Three main antipsoric remedies

1. Sulphur
2. Calcarea Carbonica
3. Silicea

The importance of Minerals as therapeutic agents

According to anthroposophic medicine, mineral substances are the most difficult to digest; and they are the farthest away from the human. A Mineral substance has to be brought back to warmth that infuses the etheric realm. Warmth is intimately related to the ego-organization. Just as the astral body is engaged with plant substance in the middle region of the human organism, so too the ego-organization is called upon to digest mineral substance in the head organization. Mineral substances can increase wakefulness as they are digested by that part of the human organism where the warmth is freed and works externally. As minerals act upon the highest level of man, the "I", they are the closest approximation to the antipsorics of Hahnemann, acting at the original source of disease, the free soul faculty of the willing of man to choose evil over good. Therefore, minerals are another homeopathic source of ultimate cure and act as a Christ impulse substance.

One of the most important mineral and antipsoric substances in homeopathy is sulphur. Shown below is the cycle of this mineral as described by Paul Herscu[93]:

Sulphur:
1. Fullness and Haughtiness: fullness in many different ways, may not just be haughtiness.
2. Sensitive to Pressure: They are so full, they hate to be overpowered; oversensitive to other people impinging on them

---

[93] Founder of the New England School of Homeopathy, Herscu is a highly recognized naturopath specializing in the study and use of classical homeopathy using his own construct of a totality known as "cycles and segments". For decades, he and his wife Amy have taught thousands of homeopaths this method of analysis which they employ in their busy practice in Hartford, Conneticut,

3. Desire to be productive: the fullness makes them want to do something to be active.
4. This leads to heating up with excitement: they become very full and active, very vibrant which leads to #5.
5. Itching: This over-heating leads to itching.
6. They scratch until the skin is damaged and discharging
7. They then become exhausted and depleted
8. They now must get away and meditate as they burn out and need to be quiet for a certain period of time.
9. As they lie there they develop ideas and start to make plans.

As shown, this is one of the warmest remedies of the "Materia Medica" and according the Rudolf Steiner, warmth is connected with the "I" consciousness. These patients are exhuberant, charismatic and tend to draw people toward them. They have ideas in abundance but their downfall is their ability to easily expend their energy resulting spending a great deal of time recharging their battery.

Calcarea Carbonica:

Calcarea Carbonica is the second most important antipsoric remedy and once again is revolved around the use and loss of a limited amount of energy to fulfil our purpose. Listed below is the cycle of this mineral.

1. weakness with slowness.
2. leads to anxiety.
3. to stop the anxiety, they need to hold back all data coming into them and categorize their reality. You will hear them repeat your instructions to slow down the information to absorb.
4. they need extra time to do things and in doing so become very busy.

5. They overwork themselves doing the work.
6. they become fatigued and shut down.

These patients can be incredibly determined people. They are very hard workers, organizing every detail, which then leads to a collapse. Sadly, they are born weak particularly in regard to processes requiring this mineral. The children are small and puny exhibiting poor development. They can be late in dental eruption and learning to walk, and are always lagging behind. They can suffer from frequent respiratory and ear infections as well as sinus trouble and heart palpitations. They tend toward constipation as a part of their overall slowness.

They have many fears especially regarding what is going to happen in the future. They are very concerned about death and they will drive people crazy with their questions revolving around this subject. They have a strong drive to truly understand things. Almost all people needing Calcarea Carbonica have a tendency to fear that they will lose their mind or develop dementia.

Change is difficult for them, especially for the children, who are only ameliorated when things are explained clearly to them. When they hear bad stories, their mind gets carried away until an explanation is given to them that makes sense.

They are happiest when they are busy until they are overwhelmed. It is at this point that they shut down. However, they desperately try not to show it to others as they worry that people might think they are going crazy or that they are inept.

This psoric remedy is chilly and slow with a strong desire to help the world. However, they choose to perform these good deeds behind the scene with no need for recognition. This is in stark contrast to the arrogance of a hot sulphur, who thrives on the challenge but collapses to a deep sleep or meditative state to begin again with enthusiasm once the proper amount of rest has been achieved.

Silicea

Like Calcarea Carbonica, this is another weak and chilly antipsoric. But unlike Calcarea this remedy is much more weak-willed and tend to take up less psychic space. Here is the cycle of this mineral

1. Weakness with a decrease in stamina. A lack of grit that results in a yielding character both emotionally and physically.
2. This causes an increased sensitivity to the things that confront them. They lose confidence as a result of being too impressionable.
3. as a result of this fear, they conform. They don't really change who they are, but conform to what people expect of them. As a result they act differently around different people depending on what that person expects. Inwardly, they do not change who they are.
4. This leads to an inflexibility. A sort of perfectionism is seen that exhibits as a concern for trifles.
5. This then causes a kind of restlessness.
6. The restlessness leads to discharges in a way that creates cracks and fissures. This results in discharges which ultimately leads back to weakness. This weakness can be seen in the mind such as comprehension and confusion.

Silicea types do not have enough to see it all the way through, including life. As a result, they need other people to help them. It plays a large role in performance anxiety and tend to be bashful and timid, even their stool is bashful. This explains its use in maturing and rupturing abscess that refuse to come to a "head" so to speak. This includes non-healing wounds and persistent fistulas.

These three remedies, along with Psorinum, are representative of a large number of remedies that are used as antipsorics. These remedies are found in their entirety in homeopathic repertories under the heading "Generalities, psora. The minerals with the highest grade of importance also include: Calcarea Phosphorica, Cuprum, Kali Carb, Mag Carb, and mag Phos.

The seven metals of anthroposophic medicine as antipsorics.

The following seven metals are considered paramount remedies in anthroposophical medicine. Although working through the etheric field, as does homeopathic remedies, these particular substances begin their effect on the all-important "I" level as explained by Rudolf Steiner. According to anthroposophical medicine, the soul faculty of weight (gravity) is reflective in strengthening of the will, also representing the soul faculty of the "I" level. The "I" level takes the healing qualities of metal and disperses it downward with the gravitational energy of metallic weight to permeate all 4 levels of the organism. The power of freeing the will (as in the term free will) allows the organism the unbounded sway of freedom to allow health at a physical level but also to achieve so much more: Promoting the freedom to create spiritually upright and correct choices toward freeing humanity and nature of the karmic debt that is the necessary cause of pain and suffering. This is the totality of spiritual science that goes far beyond the totality of Hahnemann's view of the physical-etheric-astral as the highest level of the hierarchy of man's totality. This is realized in the neuro-endocrine axis as expressed by generalities and mental symptoms.

These important metals are gold, silver, tin, copper, lead, mercury and iron. Functioning at the level of the "I", I feel they have an ability to act as major antipsorics. This is especially true if we define this word in a broader sense than the homeopathic view of an imbalance revolving around the beginning symptom of an itch. As was stated earlier, in homeopathy, pathology began with man's decision to fall from grace. That fall was the result of the weakened will (the I). Psora, in this sense, is simply the manifestation of this disease at the most basic level of a sensation or feeling. In an anthroposophical view, these metals take on different and greater qualities than they might be viewed to have in a physical proving. The problem with provings, when considering anthroposophy, lies in the lack of awareness of the effect of these metals on the 3 levels of man. In the following discussion, the metals will be examined in the light of both anthroposophic thinking and homeopathy, and the data will be assimilated to determine how to use these metals to treat patients in our care.

Silver (Argentum Metallicum) and lead (Plumbum Metallicum)

In Anthroposophic Medicine, there are 7 fundamental processes in the living organism that can fall out of balance and cause disease. Two of these processes are stabilized by the above metals. These processes are the states of anabolism (growth) and catabolism (decay). The growth process, fundamentally important in guiding the stages of development, is juxtaposed against the process of degradation or shedding such as what is seen in the process of remodelling bone and teeth. Argentum, is the metal that is used when disturbances in the fundamental process of growth is seen, while Plumbum is more involved in the shedding and decay process. These metals control all constructive phases in the organism. As such, it is logical to conclude that reproduction plays a large role in the disorders that they treat.

Argentum Metallicum (Silver)

According to Anthroposophic Medicine, Argentum controls all processes of regeneration which is controlled by the etheric body. This metal works by enhancing the connection of the etheric with the process of metabolism. Therefore, it also plays a prominent role in disturbances of intestinal reabsorption. Liquids, in particular, are not reabsorbed properly leading to the common keynote symptom of watery diarrhoea. Other symptoms would include abdominal distension, burping and other gastric complaints. Dry mucous membranes can also manifest as a symptom of this aberrant process. The result can be revealed as inflammatory lesions of the mouth and larynx. This can lead to the Argentum keynote symptom of hoarseness. In the mental sphere, Argentum dominates the cephalic pole (the brain) and as such is used for poor memory and concentration. An interesting strong rubric in Argentum patients is mind, time passes too slowly. In anthroposophic thinking, time has to do with the etheric level. The etheric level is reflected by left sided lesions which is considered a sycotic symptom in classical homeopathy. Therefore, it can be used in patients exhibiting left sided headaches. Pressure ameliorates these headaches. In AM this is explained by pressure causing an increase in consciousness. Silver also has the ability to bind the ether body to the physical. When this process is weakened, children needing this remedy will appear underweight and withered. Bed wetting with sleep walking can be included in this weakness. Also, as silver has a strong connection with the moon, the modality of "worse full moon, or moon cycle" must also be taken into consideration. In Alternative Medicine, colloidal silver is often used as an immune stimulant. In this regard, AM considers it of great value in the treatment of high fever. In a consuming fever the ether body cannot create regeneration. Another similar situation is when the patient is in shock. As viewed by Anthroposophic Medicine, the ether body separates from the physical and the astral body is "cramped" into the digestive tract. Thus, silver can correct cramping of the GI tract after a shock. As stated before, Argentum is frequently used for infertility and embryonic development due to its stimulation of the regenerative process. It can be applied to children with developmental disorders such as genital hypoplasia, and micro encephalopathy.

In classical homeopathy and its stress strain model, many of the salient features applied using the principle of A.M. can be found in the provings of this remedy. Shown below is the classical homeopathic cycle of argentum metallicum:

1. Busy doing many things (regeneration)
2. As they do more they are stimulated to do even more (over generate)
3. Start becoming stressed from doing too much
4. Collapse from stress, passing out, vertigo
5. Broken down, aging rapidly, drying up (degeneration)
6. Want to be alone and sleep, talking to them aggravates
7. Get aggravated laying down, anxiety on waking
8. Jerks, cramps and startling on sleeping and lying down
9. Get up to do things which leads back to the first step

From examining this cycle, one can see how this remedy can overlap into the regenerative tendencies as described by Rudolf Steiner. The drying up of the tissues as well as the brain as a result of excessive regeneration is a key feature of this remedy in both fields of medicine.

In Classical Homeopathy, this remedy is frequently used in neurological pain expressed as electrical, accompanied by limb jerking, particularly on falling asleep. They are full of energy but exhausted easily and take a long time to recover from any kind of exertion. As with A.M. there are many symptoms surrounding the genitalia. From a high sex drive to complete disinterest (understandable when understanding the cycle). Pathology is abundant in the ovaries and testicles. Silver targets the throat and vocal chords (silver tongued) and is the main remedy for hoarseness in speakers or singers.

Plumbum Metallicum (Lead)

Plumbum In classical homeopathy,

Plumbum is considered a very "sick" remedy and as such is more connected to the syphilitic miasm. As one would suspect, it is a very heavy remedy. The patients feel this heaviness and as a compensation for it they make noble attempts to uplift themselves. This uplifting quality may delude the homeopath into thinking they have an excess of energy. On the contrary, it is more about them squandering the little allotment they are given. With this in mind the cycle of Plumbum begins here:

1. They want to have it all to lift themselves up. Trying to feel life as they feel entitled. They try to push themselves.
2. Their bodies fall apart because They can't deal with this energy usage.
3. They then cramp up to stop the movement.
4. This cramping up Slows them down.
5. They can then Then go toward paralysis.
6. Which can then lead to atrophy or wasting of their muscles.
7. They become Discontent and resort to stimulants to get going again.

In classical homeopathy, Plumbum is often used for serious neurological diseases such as ALS. In the beginning, you will see cramping. They have difficulty expressing themselves. They feel too numb but are constantly trying to find a stimulant that will pick them back up. Their demeanour often tends to go toward haughtiness or maybe even a dissatisfaction with their lot in life. It is as if they deserved better.

Plumbum in Anthroposophic medicine

Plumbum represents death and decay; the polar opposite of the representation of Argentum. The active example of this experienced as a daily event, is the development of bone and teeth, in which living substances pass into the mineral state. This is the physiological representation of man's recognition of self. It is related to the spiritual faculty of thinking. It is said to be related to formation and consciousness through a delimiting quality as a forming impulse. This forming impulse acts through the nervous system and works right down into the mineral structures found in bone and teeth. As long as there is consciousness, aging and death will continue. Plumbum therefore represents transformation, a fitting word for this lecture as in regard to the middle treatment, Plumbum can be considered a curative agent. As this remedy has a large effect on consciousness, the consciousness won't be able to penetrate the ether body leaving one with a dulled spiritual state. Plumbum is very important in the formation and use of minerals in the body. Therefore, it is indicated in rickets. Lead, in its full material potency is a destructive poison. It's proving can affect the red blood cells, appetite and muscles. Although all nerves are included in its disturbance, the cerebral cortex is mostly involved as well as the cranial nerves that control speaking and thinking, the main attributes of the ego or I of man. Lead can also be indicated for addiction. Alcohol paralyzes the ego, disturbing the gait and speech, and releases inhibitions controlled by the ego.

Mercurius Vivus (Mercury)

Mercury in Anthroposophic Medicine

According to anthroposophic medicine, Mercury possesses the qualities of mediating and combining forces. Mercury is the messenger of the gods and as such mediates between heaven and earth, between the spiritual and the material. In healing, Mercury is seen as the "balancer" giving the excess to the deficiency. As balance is a major premise in alternative healing, this metal was dubbed the god of the physicians. It is the remedy of extremes. Mercury as a water type metal, strives for life and guides it to a higher level. This is exemplified in its antibacterial properties. Cancer is comprised of life forces that have become separated living a separate life beyond the borders of its origin. Mercury is useful as a mediator because it can not only destroy the growth but also guide it back into the original organism. This same separation from the organism occurs in nasal discharge. Using Mercury can cause the discharge to be reabsorbed.

As mentioned, Mercury can take hold of life, and as such, can destroy life with a high affinity for those processes that embrace decay, such as dental disease. It also has an affinity for the nervous system, causing tremors and eventual paralysis. Glandular structures are highly sensitive to this water metal. Congestive swellings, especially in the neck and sinus areas are particularly sensitive. A prime example is its use in the treatment of diphtheria.

As a mediator, Mercury also plays a large role in the physiology of the lung. It has been found useful in inhibiting the destruction found in bronchiectasis.

Mercury in classical homeopathy

Again, in classical homeopathy, as with most poisons, mercury would be placed under the miasm of syphilis. It is a major remedy for this Ahrimanic state. The classical homeopathic cycle is as

follows:
1. Confusion as a decrease in the ability to concentrate associated with dullness
2. This creates an unstable, chaotic thought process
3. This then leads to irrational fears (conspiracy theories)
4. They then become rigid and dogmatic in their thoughts with a tendency to become introverted
5. This isolation makes them feel threatened and over sensitive
6. They then become impulsive and even violent accompanied by even violent discharges
7. This leads to a deep depression with guilt
8. Eventually leading to a death process that is destructive as tissue decays as well as the spirit, leading to self-mutilation and even suicide

The mercury state is one of suspicion, self-loathing and destruction. The smell is putrid and the lesions are deep and destructive. As in A.M. Mercury targets the mouth, throat and ears. In the digestive symptom, the diarrhoea will be explosive. In the skin, abscesses that form will display a green discharge and will infiltrate deeper layers below the epidermis. Tremors are a common finding and a keynote for this remedy, it is often used in Parkinson's. Another keynote of Mercury is excessive salivation especially when it is accompanied by a bad smell in the mouth. There is also a large swing between two opposite states in this remedy which parallels the thinking of Mercury as a mediator in A.M.

Stannum Metallicum (Tin)

According to AM, Stannum, like Mercury is considered a metal that has a strong relationship to water. Mercury moves water, and leads it while Stannum organizes and forms it. Therefore, it is used in mucous membranes that delineate structure such as joint membranes and abdominal linings. Because of this quality, this remedy is considered by AM to be useful in pleural effusion and joint inflammation. In addition, for the same reason Stannum is also used in the treatment of glaucoma, hydrocephalus. Connective tissue and cartilage have an affinity for this metal and Tin can thus be used for the diseases of connective tissue weakness, such as tendon and spinal dysfunction. Stannum plays a strong role in Liver function. This is a logical Premise based on the fact that the liver is in a half solid state dominated by water. According to Steiner the soul faculty of will is dominated by the liver (this is also acknowledged in five element acupuncture) which when weakened can lead to depression and mania.

Cuprum Metallicum (Copper)

Cuprum in Anthroposophic Medicine

In anthroposophic thinking, Cuprum plays its most important role in transformation. This is not so much about growth as it is about growth as it is about the qualitative aspects of life. Therefore one of its main functions is in facilitating living substance into blood. It does this through the liver which is rich in copper, and at a higher level, it can allow the blood to take up soul spiritual impulses. It helps in blood deficiency states by activating ferrum in order to strengthen blood. Because of this connection, it can be used in venous thrombosis, haemorrhoids, and peripheral vascular disease. As Copper stimulates stomach acid this also helps in iron absorption.

Copper has an affinity to light which in AM is involved in the formation of pigment. In man, this is melanin and therefore can be used for such conditions as vitiligo. Copper is a very strong remedy for cramps both in A.M. and classical homeopathy. In A.M. however, the cramps are seen as a result of a weak astral body. Unable to penetrate the metabolic pole, it diverts its effect on the cephalic pole or nervous system which leads to a cramp. Copper can be used for spasms of the digestive system, the lung, and the limbs. It is often effective in the treatment of epilepsy.

Those sensitive to the world of the dead often have an untransformed astral impulse. The physical manifestation of such an abnormal connection is irritable bowel and ulcerative colitis. If both symptoms appear together in a patient, copper is often indicated.

Hyperthyroidism (Graves' disease) can also be a result of a poorly transformed Astral pulse. Copper is used to detoxify thyroxin and calm the thyroid gland.

In summary, according to A.M., copper mediates the astral body with the ether body. Physically this is manifested in the kidney.

Copper in classical homeopathy

In classical homeopathy, Copper is the only metal that is actually considered a true antipsoric. So in this case, at least, it seems to operate at the will or I level in both modalities. The cycle of Cuprum is shown below.

1. Feels various kinds of anxieties
2. Makes the patient act controlling (suppresses themselves)
3. As they close up, they get too tight
4. They need to relax
5. But relaxation makes them feel worse (vulnerable)
6. As they relax, the suppression explodes out (ailments worse rest)
7. The explosion creates a weakness with guilt, did something wrong

Studying the provings of copper reveals a strong sense of fear related to losing control. Certain provings revolve around the loss of control that causes uncontrolled entry into the spirit world. The patient will often fear or see the presence of spirits and death. This could be the proving of the weak Astral transformation of A.M. Often these patients are diagnosed mistakenly with epilepsy, which is the manifestation of an overly active astral energy. Embarrassed by the seizures these patients try desperately to regain control. So much energy is expended on this control that they have to isolate themselves from the outside stressors. As with A.M., Cuprum is the main remedy for cramping, both in the digestive system but the musculoskeletal system as well.

Ferrum metallicum (Iron)

In anthroposophic medicine, Iron is considered the metal of incarnation. In other words it is the metal that helps the spirit combine with the physical body. The higher ego body is then capable of permeating all organic processes. Though relatively unimportant in children, it becomes common in pathology relating to puberty when the iron process becomes deficient.

Iron has a significant effect on the cephalic pole especially the medulla and the subconscious. This is why it is often used in Parkinson's disease. Iron thus controls elements of coordination. Here the ego and astral body do not enter properly resulting in a loss of freedom of gait.

Iron has a strong relationship with the process of a weak bile formation. In AM this relationship results in increased activity and consciousness. If thinking is vitalized by silver, copper and mercury, formed by tin and contoured by lead, it is activated by iron. In the region of the heart it intensifies courage to be able to control himself in the world. It is the metal of the conscious soul Emotionally, ferrum relates to the anxiety created by not having enough time to do the things he needs to accomplish. This is a result of a weakened will which is compensated for by excessive ambitions and a need for work. Ultimately this fails to fulfil him and can result in a Great Depression

Classically, Iron has been used for low energy and a weakened immune system. Iron has an important role in protection against pathogens.

In this AM descriptions of ferrum there are many overlaps with classical homeopathy. The below cycle reflects such similarities

Cycle of Ferrum Metallicum (iron):

1. Anxiety of conscious about not being productive
2. Need to move
3. Strong desire to work, to fix the world, to do productive work
4. Aggravated from being interrupted, especially noise.
5. Blows up because of the interruption (see red face)
6. Followed by weakness (especially in the arms)

This is very similar to what Steiner has to say about Ferrum. The phrase "Iron will" comes to mind as a summary of this metal. With these patients there is a strong sense of guilt accompanying the frenzied work ethic. This ethic is not about money but a feeling of accomplishment. Therefore ferrum types do not like help or consolation.

Physically it has many symptoms revolving around the blood. Vertigo, head aches nose bleeds and facial flushing are all indicators of problems with circulation. Heart palpitations are common especially when accompanied by anaemia. In the stomach there is indigestions with a tendency to burp and in the lower G.I. Tract, fruits and sweets can create diarrhoea.

Aurum (Gold)

Up until now all the metals discussed played an important role in creating a balancing healthy spiritual physical being. Every metal needs to be in perfect balance. There are three polarities of the six metals that is controlled at a higher level. This control is through gold. Gold is analogous to the sun in our solar system. It is congealed sunlight to a metal substance.

All the inherent properties of the metals can be found in gold. Gold strives to harmonize and balance the polarities such as that seen in gravity and levity (material vs spiritual). Earthly forces do not affect it. Gold resists oxidation. It is truly noble in its being.

A highly psychological remedy, the gold patient tends toward a swing from mania to a severe depression with the presentation of death as to be feared and longed for. These emotional states can have a strong effect on the heart, the organ that binds spirit and body as one. Gold gives direction, it leads, it allows freedom. Again classical homeopathy has a very similar view of Aurum as shown in the following cycle

Aurum Metallicum (Gold) cycle:

1. A failure or grief happens
2. Close up as a result of that failure
3. Depression
4. Confusion of their identity
5. Guilt with suicide
6. Desires gods help to purify the soul. Hope that they will be purified
7. Anxiety leading to perfectionism
8. Work towards purity which settles the anxiety
9. More work the more arrogant the more successful
10. A grief returns that shakes your core and the cycle begins again

Aurum seek the unattainable. This leads to a deep depression that they accept as a part of the seeds they have sown. In classical homeopathy at a physical level this appears more syphilitic in nature. We find is bone destruction, ulcers in the stomach and hepatic disease. It treats many heart problems, including heart valve disease and myocardial infarction.

The metals relationship to the meridian-organ systems of five element acupuncture

Through Spiritual Science research, Are Thoresen discovered a relationship among the metals, the "planets as described by anthroposophy[94], and the meridian- organ systems of Acupuncture. These relationships are listed below:
These homeopathic preparations work against the destructive power of the Ahrimanic demons through their relationship to electricity. The symptoms created by these entities are often from the etheric body. There are 7 main metals, as there are 7 main planets that support the 7 main organs; These seven main organs are listed below

Mercurius:	Mercury	protects the intestines
Cuprum:	Venus	protects the reproductive organs
Argentum:	Moon	protects the kidneys
Aurum:	Sun	protects the heart
Ferrum:	Mars	protects the gall-bladder
Stannum:	Jupiter	protects the liver
Plumbum:	Saturn	protects the spleen

Thoresen theorizes that these remedies have a uniquely antagonistic relationship with the Ahrimanic impulse through a

---

[94] the planetary phases represent the evolutionary stages of man and the cosmos. There are 7 stages beginning at Saturn. See more aout this in chapter 28.

shared relationship to electricity. His use of homeopathy is neither classical nor anthroposophic in the traditional sense. Are uses the results of his pulse diagnosis to determine the primarily deficient meridian, and from these results administers the corresponding remedy. This is usually done using an X potency for 30 days.

Chapter 21:

Osteopathy and the Middle Point

The relationship between the middle point and osteopathy is indeed important, as this led me to find another anatomical middle-point. I invited myself to the German congress of osteopathy, held in Berlin. There I asked to give a speech and a demonstration of my new method of finding the middle or Christ point. I told the group that all osteopathic lesions could be treated by finding and treating the middle point.

For this specialized group of physicians this seemed quite outrageous. Then, as improbable as this claim would seem, the leader of the Osteopathic organization in Switzerland stood up and agreed to give it a try. She chose a patient, and I asked her to find the area of maximum excess and the area of minimum deficiency. She did so. I then asked her to "treat" just midway between the two. She questioned such a method as she was under the belief that treating a healthy spinal segment could do harm. I still asked her to treat the middle, and after some discussion she reluctantly agreed to do so. After a short time, she looked up, totally amazed. She discovered that the pathology was corrected. I had proved my new method and expected to be invited to the next year congress to present my findings to a greater audience. But I was not invited.

This method takes away all need for diagnosing, complex diagnostic procedures, and for experts. It will also take away all need for expensive courses and the need for experts. Too good to be True? I have surmised that this might be why I was not asked to come back.

Despite my "snub" by the Osteopathic society, I have seen for myself, as well as have had many colleagues confirm, that 97% of all the osteopathic lesions in horses or humans are gone after 45 minutes in a circle, treating the middle point. However, if this method was to be adopted by the osteopaths, it would mean an end to all the schools in osteopathy, a consequence that would be unsurmountable by the powers that be.

Craniosacral therapy and the Middle point

Craniosacral therapy is based on the concept that there is a subtle inherent motility of the central nervous system that can be accessed through touch, primarily at the level of the cranium and/or sacrum. The therapist lightly palpates the patient's body and focuses intently on these "movements". These small rhythmic motions of the cranial bones are used similar to the way the radial pulse is used in acupuncture. Any aberration in these movements is corrected by subtle almost etheric manipulations with a directional intention from the therapist. It seems logical, that this extremely subtle form of osteopathy lends itself to spiritual medicine.

As in all Spiritual work, we first must separate the 3 Soul Faculties (Thinking, Feeling and Willing) when we work with Craniosacral therapy. It is in this way that we use them singularly. In the body there are three cranio-sacral rhythms, one rhythm for the Etheric body, one for the astral body and one for the "I"-organization. The Etheric is stronger in the lower area of the body, the astral in the middle and the "I"-organization in the head. We must also consider that will is connected to the Etheric, feeling to the astral and thinking to the "I"-organization. We must use almost the same order and division in diagnosing. We must be in the thinking forces of the head when diagnosing the rhythm of the head. We must be in the willing forces of the earth element or the hip area when diagnosing the rhythms of the hip, digestive or reproductive system. We must be in the feeling forces of the heart when diagnosing the rhythmic system of our feeling heart and rhythmic lungs. In examining each rhythm, we must feel where the irregularities are or where there is something pathological. We then choose what rhythm to treat. In doing so, we also choose what area to treat. We also then decide whether to use the thinking, feeling or willing as a driving force in the treatment. In treatment, we use the respective forces we find in our own body. From the chest or heart we feel and use the feeling rhythm to treat irregularities in the heart rhythm. From the head we use the forces of our thinking to treat irregularities in the thinking rhythm. From the lower part of the body we use the will powers to treat irregularities of the hip rhythm and extremities.

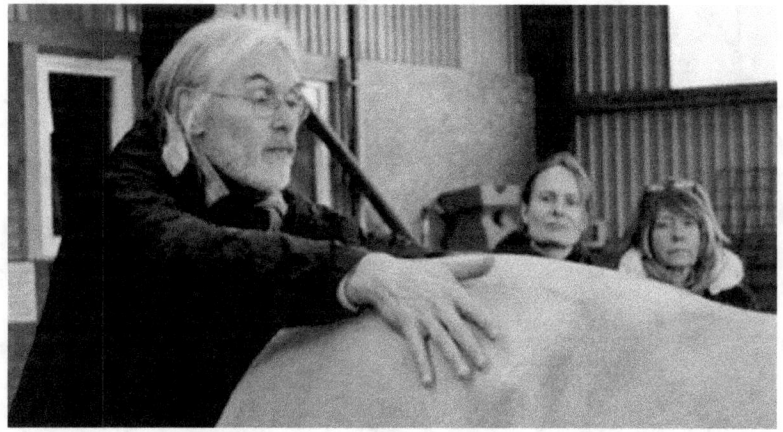

Craniosacral Therapy done on the pelvis

Chapter 22:

Closing Remarks, A Resurrection.

In my first book[95] I wrote a closing remark entitled "Requiem". The conclusion was as follows;

"We have come together in a journey of knowledge to the last page, the end of the "active life" of this book. By now, you should have spent several hours reading this work. If you have not done so, please go back and read it again before you proceed! One spoils the enjoyment of a thriller if one reads the last page first! I want you to read this requiem only when you have grasped the ideas in this book and you have made its thinking process an instinctive part of your thinking process".

A requiem is a formal farewell ceremony for the dead. In its briefest form, it can be a note on a grave, or tomb. It points beyond the grave, beyond death, to the afterlife. In the Christian tradition, the most common requiem is "Requiescant in Pacem" – "May they rest in Peace".

In a certain sense, with these last words, I want to demolish all that I have said in this book, but also show the necessity of its writing. As life that dies in the leaf fall of autumn resurrects in the green shoots of spring, this requiem shows how all that has been written in this book will resurrect in a new way, in a new life of meaning and context.

The intricate medical or healing systems that we have made and believe in, do not work in or of themselves. The most important component of healing is our own will and intention, which can kindle belief of the patient and his ability to initiate his own curative response. Most people reject the idea that an animal's "belief" (if there is such a faculty) could have anything to do with

---

[95] Holistic Veterinary Medicine, Amazon, ISBN 10-1467991104

clinical results. However, animal owners, and most good veterinarians (whether conventional or holistic) know that animals have highly developed instincts to distinguish "friend" from "foe". It is uncanny how often animals sense the good intentions of a holistic veterinarian. They usually respond by allowing handling or other interventions, such as multiple needling or spinal manipulations that would put many conventional veterinarians in great danger of being bitten, scratched or kicked! Holistic veterinarians know that animals see them as a "friend". This intention, will and courage to cure and heal, also carries the potential to heal, or start the patients self-healing abilities to cure themselves. As two of my teachers have said:

"If you can really visualize the effects of a point, you need not insert a needle" (Georg Bentze)

"If you really know the workings of a homeopathic remedy, it is enough to picture giving that remedy to the patient" (Margit Engel).

The concepts in this book are absent from, or hard to find in other books. However, these concepts are very important for professionals who want to improve their clinical success rates. When you have assimilated it and made it real for yourself, it becomes superfluous to your needs and you can dismiss it. When this happens, it resurrects as your own healing, intuitive powers. Then you become a true healer. I most earnestly invite you to try these methods with an open mind and an honest, loving heart."

In the last part of this book, centered around the soul faculty of willing, which implies the ability to "will' the correctly chosen methodology via the Christ impulse, brings this conclusion a step further. We now come to realize that death is not an end, but a beginning through the resurrection

As Christianity is nothing without the resurrection, healing is nothing without the solution of translocation. We must realize that life is spiritual, as are diseases, and translocation must be stopped through transformation. When this fundamental fact becomes part of our understanding, we become true healers.

..... **Amen**

Spiritual Medicine – A Trilogy

(On back of the book)

This book is a synthesis of four books, three published and one unpublished.

1. Alternative Veterinary Medicine (published on Amazon, Sonntag Verlag, Italian and Spanish Publishers).
2. 7-Fold way to Therapy (published on Amazon).
3. Demons – Spiritual Medicine (published on Amazon in an extensive version).
4. The Group – The Middle – The Christ (not published, incorporated as part three of this book).

Spiritual Medicine is a book written out of the certainty, knowledge and actual vision of the many Demons that surround us in our daily life and cause disease. It shares with the reader the experience of activating the middle force represented by Christ as a treatment, and revels in the knowledge of the strengthening force of the human community or Group as a force of healing.

The authors of this book have seen disease demons leave the body of the sick and enter the body of those who are not sick, thus spreading the disease (what we call contagious). We have also, in our therapeutic work, seen that the only effective way to deal with the demonic pathological entities is not to fight them, but rather to help them Transform through the boundless Love of Jesus Christ.

This knowledge is now gathered in this book, which may give the reader a better understanding of the Spiritual background of the world, of our fellow beings, of health and disease and of Angels and Demons.

We have developed a way to perceive the influence of these demons on our patients through the development of our spiritual eye (clairvoyance). This has allowed us to discover the insights leading to a beneficial treatment of the pathology that may arise from these baleful influences.

www.ingramcontent.com/pod-product-compliance
Lightning Source LLC
Chambersburg PA
CBHW052138220526

45471CB00004B/1428